Sick Business

Sick Business
The Truth Behind Healthcare in India

DR SUMANTH C. RAMAN

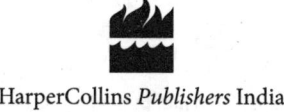

HarperCollins *Publishers* India

First published in India by HarperCollins *Publishers* 2024
4th Floor, Tower A, Building No. 10, DLF Cyber City,
DLF Phase II, Gurugram, Haryana – 122002
www.harpercollins.co.in

2 4 6 8 10 9 7 5 3 1

Copyright © Dr Sumanth C. Raman 2024

P-ISBN: 978-93-5699-725-7
E-ISBN: 978-93-5699-653-3

None of the content in this book is intended to be a substitute for professional medical advice and should not be relied on as health or medical advice, diagnosis or treatment. Always seek the guidance of your doctor or other qualified health professional with any questions you may have regarding your health or a medical condition.

The data and statistics compiled by the author is based upon publicly available information, believed to be reliable at the time of writing. Though utmost care has been taken to ensure its accuracy, no representation or warranty, express or implied, is made that such data and/or statistics is accurate or complete. Both the author and the publisher accept no liability for any loss or damage arising directly or indirectly from use of this data and/or statistics, however arising; including any loss, damage or expense arising from (but not limited to) any defect, error, imperfection, fault, mistake or inaccuracy with this book or its content.

Some names and identifying details have been changed to protect the privacy of individuals.

Dr Sumanth C. Raman asserts the moral right
to be identified as the author of this work.

All rights reserved. No part of this publication may be reproduced, stored in a retrieval system, or transmitted, in any form or by any means, electronic, mechanical, photocopying, recording or otherwise, without the prior permission of the publishers.

Typeset in 11.5/15 Minion Pro at
Manipal Technologies Limited, Manipal

Printed and bound at
Thomson Press (India) Ltd

This book is produced from independently certified FSC® paper
to ensure responsible forest management.

*To the thousands of doctors and healthcare professionals
around the country, who work tirelessly to
help lakhs of people despite all
the challenges they face.*

The detailed references and notes pertaining to this book are available on the HarperCollins *Publishers* India website. Scan this QR code to access the same.

Contents

Prologue	ix
1. Are You Being Over-tested?	1
2. Are You Being Over-diagnosed and Overtreated?	27
3. The Epidemic of Unnecessary Surgeries and Procedures	47
4. Is the Quality of Healthcare Being Measured?	65
5. Does Your Doctor Know Enough?	91
6. Patient-Centric Care	113
7. Should Healthcare Be a For-Profit Industry?	130
8. Is Big Pharma Influencing Your Treatment?	147
9. Are More Hospitals and Doctors Really the Solution?	180

10.	Public Health: The Unfortunate Orphan	203
11.	Health Insurance in India	226
12.	Can AI-supported Expert Systems Change the Face of Healthcare Delivery?	245
13.	A Doctor's Dilemma	269
14.	Navigating the Indian Healthcare System	293
	Acknowledgements	301

Prologue

I knew at an early age that a career in medicine was my calling. To my mind, there is no other profession that is as onerous and, at the same time, as rewarding as the practice of medicine. As a doctor, I have helped scores of patients. I have also lost a few along the way. Despite being in the field for over three decades, I still hurt when I lose a patient.

While I gained medical knowledge from the college, I believe that I started to truly learn about being a doctor once I started seeing patients. It is easy to memorize the symptoms of cancer in a classroom, but it is extremely difficult to deliver that news to a patient or caregiver.

There was a world of difference between theory and real life. My initial postings in government hospitals opened my eyes to the harsh realities of life. As part of the training programme, young doctors are posted to remote places for rotating internships, one of which is in a primary healthcare centre (PHC). This period is highly variable—from three months during the MBBS (Bachelor of Medicine and Bachelor of Surgery) course to two years post MBBS, if they have signed a bond with the government.

I was posted to one such PHC in Velliyur, a village not too far from Chennai but with poor commuting facilities. Doctors were expected to stay in the village and work in the PHC. There was no provision for running water at the centre, and we had to get water from a nearby well. Every day, we would have to walk to the well and fetch a bucket of water to keep outside the room for our needs, even to wash our hands between examining patients. This was the situation in the late 1980s.

This was not unique to this healthcare centre. Even today, there are many PHCs across the country without access to running water. I have also heard of many that remain locked for months, as the doctors on duty would not turn up. These doctors know the right palms to grease—they not only contrive to escape any retribution, but also to get postings at better locations.

I was told about a particular PHC in Vellore district of Tamil Nadu which was considered a difficult place to work. The doctors who were posted there had reached their wits' end and locked up the centre. But before that they had sold off some of the furniture and medical equipment and decamped from the location. It was several months before the authorities realized that the centre was not only closed but was stripped of some of the furniture and equipment.

Well into the twenty-first century, there are still many PHCs which are either completely closed or only partly functional. A few of them serve as cattle sheds and some as shelter from the elements! There is an appalling passivity when it comes to the management of primary healthcare in India.

In November 2022, a young athlete lost her life in a government hospital in Tamil Nadu due to gross medical negligence. Seventeen-year-old Priya had undergone an arthroscopic ligament repair procedure, during which a tourniquet was applied to minimize bleeding. But the hospital staff forgot to loosen the tourniquet after the surgery. When the patient screamed in pain, they gave her more analgesics to reduce the pain. They did not realize that the tourniquet had not been released and was thus effectively cutting off the blood supply to her lower limb. The prolonged pressure from the bandage caused a lack of blood flow and led to gangrene of the leg. She was then moved to another hospital, where the leg had to be amputated. However, as the treatment continued, she developed sepsis, causing multiple organ failure leading to her untimely death. A young life was snuffed out due to sheer negligence.

If you think that it is only the government sector that is apathetic, think again.

My friend and former national table tennis champion V. Chandrasekhar was admitted to one of the most well-known corporate hospitals in the country, following a recommendation, for arthroscopic surgery for a knee injury. Chandra was then only twenty-five years old, on his way to even greater heights in the field of table tennis. He went into the hospital expecting that he would, after a short rehabilitation programme, continue playing for the country. But he came out a wreck, physically. He was virtually paralysed for some time. His speech and vision were completely impaired. It later emerged that the oxygen supply to his brain was cut off during the surgery. There was a blame game between the surgeon and the anaesthetist—and though Chandra filed and won a case against the hospital much later, it was of little solace to him. A young man destined for greater heights was confined to bed for a long time and had to undergo years and years of rehabilitation programmes. Not only did his sporting career end, he also couldn't lead a normal life post-surgery. He chronicled his battles in the aptly titled book, *My Fight Back from Death's Door*. Given his celebrity status, this case made national headlines and raised a lot of public outrage. Yet, even today, there are thousands of Chandras who walk into a hospital hoping for a cure and walk out a mere shadow of their former selves. These cases are hushed up and the staff and hospital involved are rarely penalized.

If this is the state of hospitals, pharmaceutical companies are not far behind. In a country like India, medical expenses are usually out-of-pocket transactions, as not everyone is insured. Even with price regulation by the government, the cost of medication is prohibitive, and thousands of people abandon treatment midway.

For example, Trastuzumab is a drug manufactured by the Swiss pharmaceutical company Roche, and is used extensively in the breast cancer treatment. However, the drug was exorbitantly priced, costing an eye-watering ₹10 lakh for seventeen cycles of the medicine. In 2014, an Indian pharmaceutical company received approval to market a biosimilar (an affordable version of the drug). But Roche filed a suit against the company to halt the sale. After an expensive and drawn-out litigation, the Delhi High Court allowed the sale of the drug by the Indian company. There was a lot of delay before the judgement, and it is anybody's guess as to how many patients had to halt their treatment because they couldn't afford the drug.

Another area of laxity is public health. Public health policies and activities are the foundation of a healthy nation. As citizens, we assume that our elected representatives would act with our best interests in mind. The COVID-19 pandemic witnessed a vaccine race and Indians were particularly proud when our own Bharat Biotech developed a vaccine against this killer virus. But how many of us know that the company received permission for the emergency use of the vaccine without putting out trial data in the public domain? Media reports are now emerging about how the company cut corners to make the vaccine. The World Health Organization (WHO) has suspended the supply of the vaccine to United Nations (UN) agencies after investigations revealed less-than-stringent manufacturing practices.

As I spent more years in practice, I realized that the driving force behind the industry is not altruism but greed—across all levels of the hierarchy. The authorities turn a blind eye as their pockets are also lined by various players.

A study by the Public Health Foundation of India (PHFI) reveals that around 55 million (5.5 crores) Indians are pushed to poverty in a single year due to healthcare costs.[1] A few factors affecting the Indian health sector are limited access to quality care, lack of affordable hospitals, ill-equipped healthcare professionals, corporate greed leading to unwanted and unnecessary procedures, target-meeting attitudes, medicos playing God, and an almost complete lack of understanding the outcomes, consequences and management of action leading to zero accountability.

What are we doing about this? We fret and fume, hope that it does not happen to us and heave a sigh of relief if we do manage to escape the medical trap. Most of us still believe that expensive treatments at a premium corporate hospital ensures quality healthcare, and that it is only government hospitals that offer subpar treatment. We believe that if our doctor has a friendly bedside manner, they are extremely competent. But nothing can be further from the truth.

As a close witness to the many vagaries of the healthcare system, I am appalled by the general apathy and acceptance of its shortcomings. This conversation needs to take centre stage for true reform.

I am often bemused by the insouciance displayed by healthcare leaders while dealing with patients. Over the decades, I have seen a vast improvement in the quality and reach of healthcare in India. But, at the same time, I am a witness to an increased focus on profitability and an I-don't-care attitude towards patients. Many healthcare decisions are taken by people who are far-removed from the stark realities of the Indian situation. Such is the acceptance of these situations in India that, apart from a few newspaper articles and social media posts, there have been very few calls for sweeping healthcare reforms.

The Indian healthcare system, in one word, is horror. The fate of the people who enter the system depends much on God's grace and luck; it is often based on the doctor and the hospital they go to for care. I have used my personal experiences, as well as interviews and conversations with many of my colleagues and patients around the country, to highlight the sheer grotesqueness of the system. I have also used various case studies to emphasize how the system is driven by money-making motives. Through this book, I hope to make the powers be aware of how utterly inadequate we are in measuring the quality of healthcare in the country. I also recommend strategies on how we can move towards true universal healthcare, introducing compassion into our practice and always being driven by the patient's best interests and nothing else. In these efforts, I have tried to highlight some of the key emerging trends in healthcare, including healthcare technology trends that are likely to dominate the field in the coming decades.

Above all, I want to provoke your interest in a topic that affects us all.

The aim of this book is not to demean the healthcare system in India. To be fair, there are thousands of sincere, benevolent doctors and healthcare staff who put in great effort in rendering service to their patients. They are the warriors who help keep a broken and sinking system afloat, and I salute them. But they are a small minority and their well-meaning efforts are despite the system and not because of it.

This book is meant to shake you out of your complacency, to make you think deeply about the issues raised here. If it results in the improvement of the quality of healthcare delivery in India even by a fraction, then my efforts would be more than worth it.

1
Are You Being Over-tested?

If you've had a checkup done recently, it is highly probable that your doctor would have recommended a test for Vitamin D, also known as the 'sunshine vitamin'. The body synthesizes Vitamin D when we are exposed to sunlight. It is likely that you may be deficient, but you are not alone. Apparently, 70–90 per cent of the Indian population are deficient in the sunshine vitamin.[1]

Isn't it surprising to hear that almost three quarters of an entire population living in a majorly tropical country is deficient in the sunshine vitamin?

Let's take a step back. What is the average range of Vitamin D in the people of India? We do not know. Why? Because we have not defined the 'normal' range for the Indian population. We merely apply the normal range defined for the fair-skinned Western population (living in colder regions) across the entire world. What is the level of the vitamin required, below which health will be impacted in Indians? Have any studies been done to check if the so-called lower are actually normal levels in Indians? We do not know for sure. As of today, 90 per cent of Indians are diagnosed with a Vitamin D deficiency. And the treatment prescribed is to take Vitamin D supplements—which are not exactly cheap!

What we do know is that the study on the prevalence of Vitamin D deficiency in India was 'facilitated' by Abbott Laboratories, an American multinational medical devices and healthcare company which, coincidentally, sells one of the most popular brands of Vitamin D supplements in India.

Testing for Vitamin D levels was virtually unheard of in India, even as recently as two decades ago, until some marketing genius included it as a part of most 'master health checks.' There is no doubt that the scientific study on the role of Vitamin D in health and disease has greatly advanced over the last few decades and that there are serious health concerns linked to its deficiency in the Western world. But shouldn't the branding of close to a billion Indians as being deficient in a certain nutrient call for serious debate?

When Did Testing Begin?

It can be said that there are three major periods in the history of medicine.[2]

Bedside medicine, where the doctor came to the patient's house, ruled during the Middle Ages and well into the eighteenth century. As hospitals started cropping up, hospital medicine became prevalent until the nineteenth century. And then, with scientific advancements emerged laboratory medicine, which is practised till date.

Since 300 BCE, when Hippocrates examined the urine samples of patients (his way of examining the sample included tasting it!) for more accurate diagnoses, medical diagnostics have come a long way. Hippocrates is also credited with being one of the first physicians to advocate for the use of the mind and the senses as diagnostic tools. Around 180 CE emerged Galen, one of the earliest pioneers of experimental physiology. He was considered the ultimate authority in diagnosis in his era.

The tenth century witnessed the emergence Ibn Sina, a groundbreaker in medical science, whose *The Canon of Medicine* was revered as the ultimate authority of medical science till well up to the sixteenth century.

The field of medicine and physiology continued growing and each century ushered in a multitude of breakthroughs that changed the way medicine was practiced.

The twentieth century witnessed the emergence of even more sophisticated methods of diagnosis, ranging from the fields of pathology to imaging. Today, of course, technology has further enhanced these methods.

Until the early twentieth century, the microscope was considered an essential piece of equipment in a doctor's clinic. The doctors would perform most laboratory procedures themselves and arrive at a final diagnosis. It was around this time that the use of precise measurements in diagnosis increased and better laboratory techniques became more widely available. Statistical norms of the human body, both physiological and behavioural, were identified by various researchers. With the advent of hospital labs, doctors were encouraged to rely on them as an objective assessment of the patient's condition using diagnostic tests became the norm.

There was also an interesting shift in the role played by medicine in society. Before the advent of labs, doctors focused on health, or how the patient was feeling, and not on how the patient should feel or would feel a few months or years down the line. Doctors used to check for the loss of health markers due to illness, and the aim of treatment was restoring these markers. But today, doctors analyse the organs, study any deviations and set forth a treatment plan to correct the said deviation.

Nineteenth century medicine became more regulated in accordance with normality rather than with health. It formed concepts and prescribed interventions in relation to a standard of functioning and organic structure of the human body and physiological knowledge—once marginal and purely theoretical for the doctor—became established at the centre of all medical reflection.

I find this shift to be incredibly significant. This did not just affect the way the diagnostic methods were adopted by doctors, but also the way they approached the patient. Patients were told that if they wanted to stay healthy, they need to fit into certain acceptable parameters, such as cholesterol below 180, fasting glucose levels below 100, blood pressure below 120/80, etc. It did not matter if you felt fine; what mattered was what a study of your blood and bones revealed. Very often, this theory evolved because of studies which showed that among those with altered lab values, a certain percentage of them would go on to develop a disease within a period of time. That percentage may have been small, but still all those with that abnormal result get treated. Obviously, it is difficult to be sure who exactly within that small percentage would go on to develop the disease.

On the other hand, alternate medicine even today relies largely on the concept of the patient 'feeling healthy' rather than focusing on abnormal lab values.

In effect, diagnostic testing has given us an opportunity to see into the future health of the patient to arrive at a treatment decision. As a result, a patient is now treated not for a medical condition they have today but for a health issue that they may (or indeed may not) develop over a period of time. While this may be useful in reducing morbidity and mortality (though debatable in several instances), it also leads to two significant concerns:

- Clinical trials or observations of one demographic are often extrapolated to the rest of the world, as we saw in the Vitamin D example above.

- Till date, in several cases, we do not have the means to accurately identify the percentage of those who may not develop the long-term complications suggested by their abnormal lab tests. If we assume that 30 per cent of diabetics will eventually develop diabetic kidney disease, or nephropathy, this implies 70 per cent will not develop it. However, as we yet do not know for sure who that 30 per cent will be—beyond a few aspects that can exacerbate this disease, including unhealthy diet, poor control of blood sugar, lifestyle choices, etc.—we treat all diabetics with drugs to delay or prevent nephropathy. In any other industry, there would be a demand to do more studies to identify this 70 per cent more accurately and take them off medications. But in the healthcare industry, there is an incentive to keep more patients on drugs as everyone in the chain stands to gain, except the patients, of course.

The problem with diagnostic testing is that it is well established statistically that if you do enough tests, you will find at least one abnormal result. And this is even in so-called 'normal' patients who have no symptoms of ill health.

Well into the twentieth century, labs were not well-networked, and each lab determined its own 'normal' values. As the industry developed, a normal range was determined, and labs across the globe accepted these as the norm. Doctors in turn used these results to treat their patients. These ranges have changed over the years; what was previously perceived as normal is now considered abnormal as medical science has evolved and our understanding of diseases has improved. I believe that the way the normal range for a test is defined requires a complete overhaul.

Physician, Protect Thyself!

> 'If the doctor has treated a gentleman with a lancet of bronze and has caused the gentleman to die or has opened an abscess of the eye for a gentleman with a bronze lancet, and has caused the loss of the gentleman's eye, one shall cut off his hands.'
>
> —King Hammurabi, *The Code of Hammurabi* [3]

Punishment for medical malpractice is not a modern-day phenomenon, as this text from around 2030 BCE proves. However, until recently, this was more an exception than the norm. Cases would be filed only if there was a significant error of judgment or lack of care exhibited by the doctor. However, since the 1960s, the frequency of such suits has shown a marked increase, so much so that medical malpractice cases are common today—not just in developed countries, but also in the developing nations.

Another significant shift was an increase in the number of doctors. The opening of medical training centres across the world helped in training millions of students. The emergence of clinics and hospitals gave medical access to a much larger population. Simultaneously, patients also had the option of seeking medical opinion from multiple doctors.

Given all these factors, testing was soon adopted as an integral part of the clinical diagnostic process. A visit to the doctor rarely ended without a referral to a lab for further diagnosis. As the hospital industry grew, so did the medical testing industry. The number of labs grew rapidly, and hospitals and labs invested in expensive equipment as part of the process.

The Malaise of Over-testing

Testing became, then, a matter of pure economics. Let me explain this with an example of a now common test, magnetic resonance imaging (MRI)—an imaging technique that helps doctors study detailed images of tissues.

Depending on the brand, the magnetic strength and other factors (e.g., if the machine is new or refurbished), an MRI machine can cost anywhere between ₹25 lakh to ₹2.5 crore.

As a patient, depending on where you go, you may end up paying any amount between ₹2,000 to ₹15,000 for a single MRI test. If we assume that the hospital has installed an MRI machine worth ₹25 lakh and charges ₹2,000 per scan, then 1,250 patients need to be scanned to break even.

But this does not mean that all earnings after this is pure profit. The breakeven amount covers only the cost of the equipment and does not include recurring costs required for running and for the upkeep of the machine. The hospital also needs to employ skilled technicians to operate the machine and radiologists to report these scans. Obviously, all this money needs to be recovered, and what other way to do so other than to pass on the costs to the patient?

Often, doctors in hospitals are assigned 'targets', a base level of patients that they are required to refer for testing. So, what initially started as a patient-centric approach has been transformed into a bottom-line focused approach—which brings me to my bête noire, the epidemic of over-testing.

First Test and Then Consult!

Rashid* is an octogenarian, who is in reasonably good health. His daily walks, careful dietary habits and friendly nature ensured that he is physically active and mentally alert. All was well until he had a fall when he stumbled on a pebble. Though there seemed to be no other damage except for a skinned knee and palms, his son decreed that Rashid must visit the hospital. The doctor-on-call was a young physician trained at one of the best medical facilities in the country. Though a basic clinical examination did not show any indication of a broken bone or any injury to the head, and though there had been no loss of consciousness or even a history of falls on the head, Rashid was still advised to undergo a battery of tests including a CT scan to rule out a head injury.

Apart from the financial impact (Rashid was not insured), there was also an emotional impact on Rashid and his family. This was aggravated by the lab's policy of not revealing the test results to the patient. So, they had to wait to meet the doctor for the results. By the time he was given the all-clear, Rashid had been consumed by anxiety.

Hampi-based Hansika M.* shared her story with me:

'My two-year-old son was falling ill often. I initially thought that this was the usual childhood fevers and colds, but as the frequency increased, my fears also increased. I lived in a small town with no specialist paediatrician, and after many tests, the local GP [general practitioner] said that this may be an allergy and my son will grow out of it. As a first-time mother, I was not appeased. I decided to consult a specialist in one of the hospitals in the city. Little did I foresee the ordeal in store for us. It was a game of passing the parcel. We first met a paediatrician who ordered various blood tests and said that as they were inconclusive, he would like us to meet an ENT [ear, nose and throat] surgeon in another hospital. The ENT surgeon recommended additional tests, claiming that he did not trust the results of the earlier lab. I watched helplessly as my two-year old was subjected to more blood tests. As the results were still inconclusive, we were recommended X-rays and a CT scan. Have you ever tried to keep a toddler still? He made known his disapproval for the CT scan loudly and clearly! The CT scan technician then recommended that we sedate my toddler to get accurate results. After all those tests, the expert doctors said that it looks like an allergy and that my son would outgrow this phase!'

I wish I could tell you that these are isolated cases, exceptions to the rule. Unfortunately, the reality is even more shocking. In the developed world, it is estimated that up to 30 per cent of all testing may be unwarranted.[4]

In my experience and research, some of the common unnecessary tests are:

- Frequent cervical cancer screening in women
- Preoperative baseline laboratory studies prior to low-risk surgery
- Unnecessary imaging for eye disease
- Annual electrocardiograms (EKGs) or cardiac screening in low-risk, asymptomatic individuals
- Prescribing antibiotics for acute upper respiratory and ear infections
- Prostate-Specific Antigen (PSA) screening
- Population-based screening for OH-Vitamin D deficiency
- Imaging for uncomplicated low back pain in the first six weeks
- Preoperative EKG, chest X-ray and pulmonary function testing prior to low-risk surgery
- Cardiac stress testing
- Imaging for uncomplicated headaches

Have you ever been asked to get these by your medical provider?

Are Tests Infallible?

I have an example closer to home.

My father went in for a 'routine' health checkup and the results showed slightly elevated levels of alkaline phosphatase (ALP), an enzyme found in the body. There were no symptoms, and he was perfectly healthy otherwise. But I reviewed the test results as a son, and not as an impartial doctor. I spoke to other colleagues—experts in this field—and subjected my father to multiple follow-up tests including bone scans. We must have spent almost ₹25,000 just on the tests. My father's stress levels increased with every test and that affected his overall health. Nothing was found and I was told that this slightly elevated level could be ignored. After years of repeated tests, I finally realized that these levels were normal for him, and it did not require any further intervention. If this could happen in my home, with all my medical know-how, what hope is there for families with little or no education?

Don't get me wrong—testing is absolutely necessary and has transformed the way medical science now manages diseases. Testing has greatly helped reduce morbidity and mortality for a multitude of conditions. But we are now at a stage where testing is often done for reasons other than the best interests of the patient. And that has to stop.

Let us re-examine the concept of the 'normal range'. For example, a hundred people undergo a routine blood test to measure levels of fasting blood sugar. The global 'normal' is less than 100 mg/dL (5.6 mmol/L). Normal ranges are calculated based on the 95 per cent confidence interval, that is, in a given population, 95 per cent would be expected to fall within that range. On any day these tests were administered, five out of the hundred will fall outside this range. These five may not have any other symptoms and the results may have been an aberration. But human nature being what it is—there would also be multiple other tests—the increased stress levels alone may elevate many factors in the human body! When asymptomatic people are tested, the chances of false positives are higher.

False Positives and Negatives

Sometimes, test results can be faulty. They may either be a false-positive (the results indicate erroneously that you have that disease) or a false-negative (you have the disease, but the test results indicate otherwise). Both these scenarios are scary. The former leads to unnecessary stress and emotional upheavals and the latter lulls you into a false sense of security. A few of the reasons for an abnormal test result include:

- Sample collection errors
- Errors in sample transportation
- Errors in sample processing in the lab
- Variations within the individual that are difficult to explain—patients sometimes have an isolated abnormal lab value
- An actual disease or pathological state in the patient

Axiomatically, only the last of these is significant for the patient.

Dr Rajendra Badwe and Dr Sudeep Gupta, the director and deputy director of Tata Memorial Hospital respectively, are arguably the final word in cancer treatment in India. They stated in an article published in *South Asian Journal of Cancer*,[4] 'Screening mammography has substantially increased the number of early-stage breast cancer cases, only marginally reduced advanced stage presentation, resulted in substantial overdiagnosis, and has had little or no effect on population breast cancer mortality.' They further say, after conducting randomized trials with over 6 lakh healthy women, 'The practical interpretation of these statistics is that the cancer in one out of three to four women diagnosed though screening mammography would either never have surfaced during their remaining lifetimes or only after a couple of decades of the mammographic label.'

Take a minute to ruminate over this. If a hundred women were diagnosed, almost twenty-five of them may never develop cancer or may develop it after decades of screening. But because of the results, these women live lives with a proverbial sword hanging over their heads. The stress in turn creates other health issues and they end up living suboptimal lives.

Another example is the exercise stress test. This test is supposed to indicate how your heart will react in stressful situations and whether you could have cardiac ischemia. While this is a useful test if you are symptomatic, there is enough anecdotal evidence that shows doubtful results are generated even if the person is asymptomatic. There are enough studies that reveal increased stress testing has led to an increase in angiography procedures and in the rate of stenting. However, there is no change in the rate of myocardial ischemia. Isn't that ironic?

Exposure to Unnecessary Radiation

Have you ever wondered why the technician wears protective clothing and leaves the room when you go in for an X-ray? Simple—to prevent exposure to radiation! Why? Because exposure to radiation increases the risk of cancer, the emperor of maladies. Be it a CT scan or an MRI, many imaging tests deliver some amount of radiation in one form or another (MRI does not deliver ionizing radiation but delivers electromagnetic radiation). Every time a patient is referred for an imaging test, it increases the risk factor.

The Numbers Don't Make Sense

We live in the age of preventive medicine, which aims to prevent the advent of disease before it becomes fatal. Vaccines are a great example of preventive medicine—they have eradicated many deadly diseases and have considerably improved the quality of life of millions. In the same vein, we have many screenings that help prevent (or result in early care for) serious health issues ranging from cancer to heart ailments. This is now becoming a multibillion-dollar industry which operates on fearmongering. Every day, we are bombarded by messages adjuring us to do such and such tests to help us detect the issue early. It doesn't matter if you are in the at-risk group or not. We have blanket statements like, 'All women must have an annual pap-smear', 'Everyone must have an annual physical examination', 'All men over a certain age must test for PSA', 'Everyone over a certain age must test for cognitive issues.'

The financial implications are also high—irrespective of who pays for the tests.

Why Do Doctors Over-test?

Based on my experience and interactions with colleagues, I collated a few reasons as to why doctors over-test. Each of these is preceded with comments from doctors I spoke with, and their names have been changed to respect their privacy.

Inexperience, lack of knowledge or confidence

In the words of Dr Tarun Irani,* a physician from Noida, 'Despite the gruelling training we endure as doctors, it is still difficult for us to always maintain our equilibrium—especially when we are new to the field. I remember my days in the emergency room. There would be days when we would be swamped with cases, and I would have to manage a few of them on my own. I would order a few tests just to buy some time—even if I was unsure that they were not really essential. Also when I could not make a diagnosis the hope was that the tests would show the way forward'.

Like all other industries, medicine is highly competitive, and very few doctors want to appear to be lacking in knowledge before their peers. These doctors then tend to practice defensive medicine by referring their patients for diagnostic tests.

Another reason why younger doctors may tend to order more testing is that their training may have been more testing focused as compared to their older colleagues, who were taught more clinical skills. There is enough anecdotal evidence which show how old GPs would diagnose a condition just by clinical observation, and this would later be corroborated by diagnostic tests.

Doctors must know their own limitations and ask for help or follow well-defined protocols if they are unsure about what to do, rather than subjecting patients to a series of tests.

Profit motive

This is Dr Vimla Yadav's* story. The orthopaedic from Nainital recounts, 'I have always wanted to be a doctor as I believed that this was a very noble profession. I worked hard throughout my years of schooling and consistently achieved good grades and qualified for admission in a prestigious medical institute. My father was a millworker, and we did not have the financial bandwidth to pay the fees. He mortgaged the house, borrowed from moneylenders, and managed to pay. By the time I finished my specialization in orthopaedics, the interest on the borrowings had ballooned and moneylenders were making threatening calls. It was then a medical lab approached me with a proposal: I refer patients to the lab, and they give me a percentage of their earnings. The more expensive the tests, higher the earning potential! Within a year, I had managed to pay back the borrowed money and by the next year, I paid back the mortgage too! And all I had to do was just refer patients for tests.'

One of the top reasons for over-testing is definitely the incentives offered to doctors for ordering tests. A test must be ordered for a patient ONLY and ONLY if it will benefit the patient, or if not doing it will cause harm. Any other reason is a corruption of the Hippocratic oath that doctors take. In many countries, doctors make as much money through kickbacks from labs, imaging centres and even referral hospitals as they do from their own practice. This practice is so rampant that it is difficult to monitor.

What first starts as a strategy to recover the investment and maintenance costs catapults to never-ending greed. This greed has also given rise to sink-testing, where the lab literally pours down the collected samples down the sink and generates fabricated results. This grim practice is common in countries where the health sector is highly corrupt and poorly regulated. The nexus between the political powers, businesspersons and medical practitioners definitely does not have the patient's best interests at heart.

In most cities and towns in India, 'referral charges'—a euphemism for kickbacks—can be as much as 25 per cent of overall patient spending.[5] Ever wonder why a doctor insists on a certain lab or a testing centre? And why the MRI scan of the brain costs ₹6,000 there as compared to ₹3,500 at another centre? It is mostly about kickbacks, though in some cases there may be genuine concerns about quality too. The labs and centres return the favour by paying the doctors in cash—stuffed into plain white envelopes and door delivered to them each month; perfect for tax evasion!

Another reason is pressure from the hospitals where the doctors work. Most of the corporate hospitals have in-house labs and imaging facilities. These hospitals set revenue referral targets for doctors, which is reviewed periodically by the management team. To protect their jobs, medical professionals are forced to meet these targets.

Unexpected diagnoses

'Yuvraj* and his family have been my patients for the past decade or so—nothing chronic or critical. He would see me for seasonal flus and the occasional stomach infection. His young daughter would see me more often for the usual litany of childhood complaints. As a family, they were health-conscious and since we moved in the same social circles, I would play the occasional round of tennis with him. He did everything in moderation, and I would say that he was a perfect specimen for a forty-five-year-old male. As a part of some financial investment decisions, he was referred for some routine medical tests—the usual blood work and stress test, etc. His test results revealed a few abnormalities, and after further testing, he was diagnosed with multiple myeloma. He was gone within six months! I still cannot believe that I missed the signs. I now refer all my patients for testing—more for the sake of my mental stability,' reminisces Dr Piyush Dugad,* a GP from Udaipur.

As doctors, this not an isolated example. All of us have had patients who looked 'normal' and then suddenly developed complications. These cases of unexpected diagnoses encourage many of us to resort to over-testing. We lose confidence in our abilities and start practicing defensive medicine. This also protects us if we are dragged to the court by patients.

Patient 'experts'

The Gurgaon-based GP Dr Anjali Sengupta recounts,* 'I remember this patient who walked into my clinic—she was around thirty-eight years old, and she wanted a thyroid scan. I suggested that we first do an ultrasound and, if needed, we can do the scan later. But she insisted that she needed a thyroid scan as she had read an article on the internet which recommended it for anyone with what looked like a lump in the neck. I tried counselling her and explaining why my medical training and experience makes me a greater authority on this topic, but she refused to listen. She said that if I would not write the recommendation, she would go to another doctor!'

Dr Aarav Desai,* an Ahmedabad-based GP, has had similar experiences. 'I find it increasingly difficult to manage patients. Even ten years back, I did not face this challenge. Today, I have patients walking into my consultation room and telling me what is wrong with them and what are the tests I should be writing up for them. And what is even more frustrating is that none of them have any medical qualifications or are even remotely connected to the field. How would they like it if I enter their workplace and tell them how to do their job? I gave up the fight and now just write up whatever tests they want. I can spend that time treating people who really need my expertise!'

In all fairness, I cannot lay the blame solely on the medical profession. The last decade has seen a dramatic increase in the number of people who are certified by the ubiquitous 'Dr Google'. People believe that the medical profession is out to 'get them', and that their doctor does not know anything and is mostly out to milk what they can from their patients. They pressurize us to refer them to tests till we find it easier to give in!

Do We Really Need a Master Health Checkup?

I recall my schoolmate Ashok's* case. Five years ago, I got a call from him. He sounded visibly agitated as he said that his thirty-year-old brother, Ravi,* was scheduled for a regular coronary angiography and the doctors had asked them to be prepared for a possible angioplasty. Ashok wanted my opinion on the hospital and the doctors. The hospital was one of the new corporate hospitals in the city and I knew the investors by reputation. I was more concerned about the young man. I had last seen him at a party, and he looked healthy: he was not overweight, was a non-smoker and exercised regularly. I also knew that Ashok did not have a family history of heart diseases. As I questioned further, the story came out. Ravi was asked to go in for a health checkup as part of the recruitment protocol for an IT company. There was a slight aberration in his stress test. The doctors then recommended a thallium stress test, which was normal. But 'just to be sure', they also recommended a 320-slice CT coronary angiography, which was inconclusive. And now, they were recommending a regular coronary angiogram 'to put all doubts to rest'.

All this in a healthy thirty-year-old man! His other health markers were normal. Now, the stress test is no longer recommended as a diagnostic test in the US and other developed countries. But it is exceedingly common in all corners of India.

The annual or master checkup was started as a screening test to help doctors nip problems in the bud. Early detection and early treatment were its mantras. As hospitals became increasingly profit-oriented, the master checkup was advertised heavily and millions of asymptomatic people adopted this regime 'just to be safe'. What started as a few basic tests quickly ballooned into additional testing. One of the most reputed diagnostic companies in the country offers an impressive health checkup package comprising of 133 tests! Most of these tests are completely unnecessary and useless. This checkup includes testing for toxic elements in the blood—most of these levels are rarely found to be abnormal in the population. But, as I mentioned earlier, statistically, five out of a hundred people will fall in the abnormal range. Most doctors have no clue what to do when a patient has a slightly elevated vanadium or molybdenum level (yes, some master health checkups do routinely screen for heavy metals; dozens of them). Another issue is tests being ordered in groups and repeated the same way. For example, in a complete blood count, most doctors hardly look at the results of all the tests it covers.

Routine ultrasounds for the abdomen are not recommended in any developed country, but in India, it is the holy grail of testing. This throws up results of fatty livers or small renal or ovarian cysts (in women), which are not life-threatening and generally do not need any medical attention. However, how many of us can live with this thought once a doctor has flagged an abnormality in our body? As Mahatma Gandhi said, 'Fear of disease killed more men than disease itself!' Only and only if there is conclusive evidence that early detection and intervention result in reductions in morbidity and mortality from a disease should the test or procedure be recommended.

Are We against All Screening Tests?

I am certainly not against diagnostic testing. Medical testing has been and will remain one of the most effective diagnostic methods. If you are diabetic, you must have your regular medical tests as prescribed by your attending doctor. In this case, regular testing for levels of blood sugar and HbA1C is an integral part of the treatment plan. But if you are not diabetic and have no genetic disposition and have a healthy body weight and lifestyle, then you may not benefit from six-monthly testing, unless you display any symptoms.

> The WHO has defined criteria for evaluating population-wide screening tests, which may help you decide whether or not to have such a test. The WHO criteria include the following:[6]
>
> - Screening should be done only for diseases with serious consequences, so that screening tests could potentially have clear benefits to people's health.
> - The test must be reliable enough, and not harmful in itself.
> - There must be an effective treatment for the disease when detected at an early stage, and there has to be scientific proof that treatment is more effective when started before symptoms arise.
> - Neutral information should be made available to the public to help people decide for themselves whether or not to have a screening test.

The WHO points out that detecting a disease early does not automatically have a benefit in all cases. If early diagnosis and treatment does not lead to an improved health outcome, early detection only makes people worry and undergo treatment for longer.

What Is the Solution?

It is time for doctors to rethink the way they test. It is time for us to go back to basics of clinical diagnosis before blindly referring patients for diagnostic tests.

Healthcare always follows the safety-first and zero-risk approach. As a patient, that is what you would want for yourself too. Every patient wants to be completely sure that the abnormal value from their checkup is not significant. It then follows that you would not be averse to undergoing more follow-up tests. Doctors cannot be blamed too—as, in many countries, they could face a malpractice suit if they did not follow up on an abnormal test that later turned out to be significant. Hence, asking doctors not to follow up on isolated, mildly abnormal tests is not the answer.

> The golden rule? As doctors, ask these questions before we order the tests:
>
> - Will ordering this test help me in making a diagnosis?
> - Will ordering this test be necessary to correlate other test results that have already been deemed essential to help confirm a diagnosis?
> - Will the test result have an impact on my treatment plan?
> - Does the test result have any bearing on the prognosis for the patient?

- Will not doing the test have any impact on the clinical outcome or patient morbidity and mortality?
- If the answer is no to at least one of these questions, then there is little reason to order the test.

2

Are You Being Over-diagnosed and Overtreated?

Back in January 2017, my colleague's father, Krishnan,* had a disturbing episode where he displayed erratic behaviour. Naturally, my colleague and her family were worried and consulted a highly-recommended neurologist in Hyderabad. On examination, the neurologist did not find anything wrong apart from age-related issues. He referred them to his colleague, a consultant psychiatrist. My colleague recounts, 'It was the most horrific time. The doctor kept shooting questions to my father as if it was a cross-examination. The questions were asked rapidly, and my father, who was already tired from the long drive and wait at the hospital, couldn't answer them instantly. I suggested that we come back another day when my father was a bit more rested. The doctor shot down this suggestion and announced that it was the start of Alzheimer's. You can imagine our shock. The doctor then proceeded to prescribe Donep-M twice a day. We immediately started the treatment, and within a few days, my father's condition deteriorated. He even forgot if he had eaten, and his daily routine went for a toss. We were scared and started researching care homes, etc. After a week of this behaviour, I reached out to another neurologist who said that Donep-M is never a first line of treatment and asked to bring my father in for a consultation. It turned out that my father was just super anxious about his general age-related health issues, which led to an emotional breakdown. This doctor prescribed a mild anti-anxiety pill and recommended exercises and some vitamins. Today, at eighty-two, my father is active and very much alert mentally.' She went on to add, 'This dangling sword of Alzheimer's affected the entire family and my mother developed health issues post this episode. I wish I could name and shame the doctor and take him to court. But, considering the Indian legal system, it may be decades before we get any relief. It is just not worth it.'

As the second wave of COVID-19 shook the country, every day brought in some fresh hell. Take the example of Arun Vijay,* a thirty-seven-year-old expat living in the US, who recounts, 'Those months were horrible. Whenever my phone pinged, my stress levels would shoot up. And, sure enough, it would be the news of one more family member dying, hospitalized or suffering from severe symptoms even after weeks of infection. I have never felt so helpless in my life!' Many like him are still struggling with the aftermath of the pandemic.

At the start, the anti-malarial drug Hydroxychloroquine (HCQ) was heavily recommended as a treatment for COVID-19. This was soon disputed by the US and UK regulators after randomized clinical trials showed no tangible benefit against the virus. The WHO issued a directive discouraging the use of HCQ as a treatment for COVID-19. But the Indian Council of Medical Research (ICMR) issued a directive endorsing its use. It took major pushback from many doctors and members of the public for prescription numbers to come down. In many cases, patients were overtreated, which potentially caused harm. Much attention has been drawn to the early use of steroids for COVID-19 treatment that could have actually increased the severity of the disease in many patients. Likewise, it is believed that the overenthusiastic use of steroids led to patients being infected with black fungus, resulting in death in several cases. Of course, as a medico myself, I understand why doctors would want to overtreat in such cases. We are trained to do something, not just wait and watch. We are trained to use whatever weapons we have in our arsenal and attack the disease, with all guns blazing. So, to sit and watch the macabre dance of the disease is unacceptable to us. But what we need to understand is that overtreatment can often be more damning than taking no action at all.

What Is Overtreatment?

In the strictest terms, 'overtreatment' refers to unnecessary medication or surgical procedures. But broadly, it can be defined as the treatment of a condition or symptom that would have otherwise mitigated with time or will not cause any significant harm to the patient if left untreated. Overtreatment falls under the umbrella of unnecessary healthcare. This can mean extra diagnostic procedures, avoidable surgeries or the practice of polypharmacy—the usage (often unnecessary) of multiple medicines in patients. For the sake of this book, I use it as an umbrella term to refer to the practices of defensive medicine, overuse of medicines, overdiagnosis and over-prescription. Normally, overtreatment is the after effect of over-screening and overdiagnosis.

Let me give you a few examples of overtreatment.[1]

Arthroscopic surgery is often recommended for mild to moderate knee osteoarthritis. But a well-designed randomized controlled trial proved that arthroscopic surgery was no more effective than sham surgery (when the patient is operated but no actual surgical procedure is done internally) for cases with mild to moderate osteoarthritis of the knee.

In the recent past, diabetes has become very common. One of the reasons for this is the recommended HbA1C (a common test to diagnose prediabetes and diabetes, it measures the average blood sugar levels over the past three months) targets being below 7 per cent, especially for middle-aged and older patients. However, three large trials found no benefit or increased mortality rates with more aggressive HbA1C targets.

There has also been an increase in surgical treatment of low-grade prostate cancer. However, Prostate Cancer Intervention Versus Observation Trial (PIVOT) found no survival benefit for surgery compared to watchful waiting.

I see a definite increase in medication and treatment of pre-hypertension and mild hypertension. But a Cochrane review found no reduction in cardiovascular events such as heart attacks with treatment of mild hypertension.[2]

Often, a vertebroplasty is recommended for painful vertebral compression fractures, even though two high-quality randomized controlled trials found no benefits that saline injections couldn't provide.

Newer diagnostic methods and the unchecked use of screening tests lead to diagnoses that otherwise may have been missed. While newer diagnostic methods were initially touted as a good thing, medicos soon realized that this is a double-edged sword. We are diagnosing probable diseases and hence are forced to treat them—even if the patient is asymptomatic. Often, the treatment is more damaging and leads to multiple complications. The data below shows how some common diseases face the brunt of overdiagnosis.[3]

> Asthma: 30 per cent of diagnosed persons may not have asthma and 66 per cent may not even require medication
>
> Breast cancer: One-third of screening-detected cancers may be over-diagnosed.
>
> High cholesterol: Up to 80 per cent of patients with mild elevation of cholesterol levels are cases of overdiagnosis.
>
> Lung cancer: Twenty-five per cent of screening-detected lung cancers represent overdiagnosis.

Another reason for this is reclassifying or redefining the thresholds of diseases. A threshold is the medically acceptable level of the parameters that are being measured. For example, haemoglobin levels between 14 to 18 g/dl and 12 to 16 g/dl are considered normal for males and females respectively. Over the years, these levels have been changed by health authorities for various reasons, ranging from increased complications because of a particular ailment to overcautious authorities to sheer pressure from the pharma nexus.

> A 2016 publication by Jaimin R Bhatt and Laurence Klotz[4] reveals that with the threshold of fasting glucose changing from 140 to 126, there has been increase in diagnosis of diabetes by 14 per cent. Similarly, there was a 35 per cent increase in the diagnosis of hypertension after a change from 160/100 to 140/90. Lowering total cholesterol threshold from 240 to 200 saw a whopping 86 per cent increase in hyperlipidaemia diagnoses. These thresholds have further changed. At the time of writing this book, the acceptable thresholds are 100 for fasting glucose, 180 for total cholesterol and 120/80 for hypertension.

Let us look at some of the diseases where overtreatment is common, and its consequences on patients, families and the healthcare system.

Overtreatment in cancer

The word 'cancer' always spreads dread amongst people; 'As long as it is not cancer, it is okay,' is a commonly heard refrain among families. Cancer has also played a leading role in many popular movies, with the protagonist eventually succumbing to the disease after reels of heart-wrenching pathos. It is one of the leading causes of death in the world. But all cancers do not cause death. People have been known to live with undiagnosed 'cancer' with no trouble and die of something totally unrelated. For example, most patients who have been diagnosed with prostate cancer after the age of seventy-five die of other causes and not of the cancer itself, even as the cancer grows slowly. We have witnessed a spike in aggressive screening tests for various types of cancers in the last few decades. This has led to an increase in the diagnostic numbers, especially in the number of indolent cancers, which are cancers that grow so slowly that they are unlikely to cause any harm in the lifetime of the individual. According to oncologist Dr Feroz Ahmed,* 'Not all cancers are alike. And not all cancers require an all-guns-blazing treatment approach. In fact, aggressive treatment of indolent cancers often causes more harm than good. Screening and diagnostics are not cheap and if there is even a slight suspicion of anything amiss, the patients are asked to repeat the tests. The financial stress, psychological stress, unnecessary exposure to radiation—they are sometimes just not worth it. The irony is that while there has been a drastic increase in the number of diagnoses, there is no proportionate decrease in the rate of deaths due to cancer.'

One of the 'cancer survivors' we spoke to, Kasturi Nair,* says bitterly, 'I don't know if I am a cancer survivor or a diagnosis survivor. It was one of those "master checkups for women" and I walked in feeling fine and healthy. I walked out with a breast cancer diagnosis (ductal carcinoma in situ, or DCIS), and I was immediately referred to the hospital oncologist. I had no time to think. I was all numb and the words "cancer" and "death" kept playing in my mind. I had no family history of cancer. The oncologist suggested a lumpectomy followed by an aggressive chemo and radiation treatment. I agreed as I knew that cancer needed harsh measures. What followed was sheer agony. I wouldn't wish it on my worst enemy. It was only much much later, when I attended a support group, that I understood I might not have needed such aggressive treatment in the first place. In cases like mine, where there is no genetic history, a lumpectomy followed by a wait-and-watch approach with close monitoring may have sufficed. Chemotherapy is not routinely indicated. But it is too late for me. I lost my health, my money, my job. Now, I am a patient advocate and I tell everyone to get a second opinion before starting with any form of aggressive treatment.'

Overtreatment in hypertension

Hypertension, or high blood pressure (high BP), is rated as one of the most common causes of death globally. In India, it is estimated that it contributes to around 57 per cent of all stroke deaths and 24 per cent of all coronary deaths. Recent studies reveal that almost 25 per cent of the urban population and 10 per cent of the rural population suffer from hypertension.[5] While these numbers are alarming, how many of these people actually need treatment for the disease? Take the case of Rajesh Vaidya,* a thirty-six-year-old sales executive. His BP remains consistently above 140/90 over a month of monitoring. He is pre-diabetic, has elevated cholesterol levels and is overweight. His job as a sales executive means that he doesn't have a regimented diet nor does he exercise. He has irregular sleep patterns too. To avoid future complications, he must be put on antihypertensive drugs.

His father, Sanket Vaidya,* is a seventy-five-year-old retiree who lives in a small town. He has a daily exercise routine, watches what he eats and is not overweight. His medical reports are absolutely fine; he is non-diabetic and has no other medical issues. Once, he was admitted to the hospital after a fall. When he was admitted, he had a BP reading of around 160/100. During a week's stay, his BP varied between 130/90 to 150/90. When he was discharged, along with his pain medications, he was prescribed an antihypertensive drug. Even after he recovered from his fall, he complained of fatigue and listlessness. He transformed from an agile, alert senior to a morose and grumpy old man. It was not until they took a second opinion from another doctor did they realize that the BP medicines were the culprit. The reason for the high BP in the hospital was the stress caused by the pain post his fall. The attending doctor, instead of waiting and monitoring his BP post-discharge, was quick to prescribe medication.

Antihypertensive drugs used in the treatment of adults (primary prevention) with mild hypertension (with a systolic BP of 140–159 mmHg or diastolic BP of 90–99 mmHg) have not been shown to significantly reduce mortality or morbidity in randomized controlled trials. Nine per cent of patients discontinued treatment due to adverse side-effects.[6] We need a more judicious approach to managing mild hypertension, especially if the person does not have other comorbidities.

Over-prescription of antibiotics

Who amongst us haven't been prescribed antibiotics at one time or the other? They are one of the most important weapons in a doctor's arsenal to fight bacterial infections—not only in humans, but also in animals. Over decades, India has emerged as the antibiotic capital of the world because of the rampant overuse across the nation. Antibiotics are often prescribed for conditions where they are not needed. For example, the first and second waves of COVID-19 in the country saw a huge increase in the sales of antibiotics. This, despite the fact that antibiotics cannot treat a virus. We may never know the percentage of morbidity or even mortality that occurred due to the inappropriate use of antibiotics.

Hubballi-based physician Dr Apeksha Mann* says, 'I have recently started my own practice as a general physician in a small town. Every day, I have at least five patients who insist on an antibiotic prescription. A few of them understand when I explain why it is not recommended in their case. But others just go to another doctor and spread negative reviews about my practice. I don't know how long I can hold on to my principles.'

Recently, a friend called to say that he had three episodes of diarrhoea since that morning. He had no other symptoms and was eating normally with no abdominal pain, fever or vomiting. I reassured him that he would be fine and told him to hydrate himself and wait until the evening. But being an anxious person, he called up another doctor within the next two hours. He then sent me a photo of a strip of Norfloxacin and Tinidazole combination that the doctor had asked him to take for three days. This was prescribed without the doctor even seeing the patient. These medicines are not recommended for viral diarrhoea and can even cause harm in some patients.

Antimicrobial resistance has been recognized as one of the top ten global public health threats by the WHO. Unlike non-infectious diseases, antibiotic-resistant bacteria can spread to anyone and is not limited by boundaries of geography, economic status, age group etc. We are at a point when virtually all significant bacterial infections in the world are becoming resistant to the antibiotic treatment of choice. For some of us, bacterial resistance could mean more visits to the doctor, a lengthier illness and possibly more toxic drugs. For others, it could mean death.

Antibiotic overuse in treating animals also increases resistance in humans. Consumption of animal products and direct contact with livestock can spread resistant bacteria to humans. While there are laws to regulate usage of antibiotics, without strong enforcement, there will be no end to bacterial mutations resulting in superbugs that can kill.

How Does Overtreatment Start?

When do we go to see a doctor? This seems a simple enough question but think a bit and you will find that the answer is not so easy. The logical answer to the question would of course be that we go to a doctor when we are sick. Think again: do we go when we are sick or when we feel unwell? Obviously, the answer is the latter as being 'sick' would mean knowing the disease, but we are not qualified enough to know if we have a definitive identifiable—one which can be diagnosed conclusively by a physical examination or a lab diagnostic—disease or not. So, when we feel unwell, we go to a doctor.

In my experience, 35 per cent of patients who attend outpatient clinics for a consultation either have no definitive identifiable organic illness or have a condition that may require only symptomatic treatment. Many of them may require no treatment at all. This includes the large number of patients with self-limiting conditions. Yet, all these patients need to be looked at by the doctor, who then needs to assess if the patient falls into a category that needs further investigation or indeed if the symptoms may be due to an organic illness. Almost all the patients will receive some medication, and many of them will be put through tests to ensure they do not have any organic illness. This effectively means that close to a third of the patients that doctors around the world are 'treating' have no definitive illness.

In any other industry, the odds of this happening would be very low. For example, when your car does not start, it is because there is always a problem. It may be a minor issue like a loose battery wire or a major problem like a self-motor failure but always because there is a problem that needs to be attended to—in other words, the car cannot 'feel' that it does not want to start without anything being wrong. However, in humans, that is obviously not the case. Thousands of depressed patients and those with psychosomatic illnesses visit clinics for some ache or pain that has no identifiable cause. They receive the same level of initial attention from the doctor as those with definitive organic illnesses. All of them receive some level of medication and many of them have at least a few tests done.

It is apparent that doctors spend as much of their time in ascertaining patients have no illness as they do in treating those who do. For the private sector, this works just fine. After all, the patients who have no significant illnesses are easier to treat as most of them will get better anyway and they also add to the revenue of the hospital and doctor. For the government, though, it is a huge problem. As any doctor working in a PHC in India will attest, they could do a much better job at managing their patients if they had to see fewer numbers each day. According to my assessment, the average time spent by a doctor in a PHC, diagnosing and treating a patient, is around three minutes or less. This includes the time to write out the prescription. It is absurd to expect that in three minutes a doctor will be able to identify all the relevant symptoms, take a detailed history and carry out a preliminary examination on the patient as well as write out the prescription. In practice, what happens is that the doctor asks the patient to list their symptoms and, based on their duration and severity, the prescription is dispensed. The doctor may place a stethoscope on the patient or palpate an abdomen but there is hardly any time to carry out a detailed examination. In some cases, doctors even prepare the prescription slips in advance. There would be a 'myalgia' prescription for patients with body ache, which would include B complex (BCT) or multivitamin tablets (MVT) along with paracetamol; for lower or upper respiratory infection prescription, you'd get an antibiotic with an antihistamine and paracetamol and so on. The appropriate drug slip would then be given after writing the patient's number on it. This is what happens in many PHCs around the country. To be fair, it is not the doctor's fault. They need to see on average sixty to seventy patients—in many cases more than a hundred—in a three-to-four-hour time frame. In this scenario, the truly ill patient with pneumonia and the one who has 'myalgia' get the same time and attention from the doctor. The odds of the pneumonia being missed or misdiagnosed as a mere lower respiratory infection (LRI) are much higher because

How Does Overtreatment Affect You?

the doctor just does not have the time to carry out a detailed examination.

As I mentioned earlier, the primary reason for overtreatment is overdiagnosis. Doctors arrive at a diagnosis based on the results of screening tests and not on symptoms, labelling otherwise healthy individuals as patients. This leads to severe psychological distress—not only in the individual, but also in their social cohort.

The problem often starts with master health checkups or full body health checks. When dozens of unnecessary 'screening' tests are done, the probability of one or two results being marginally off the normal range increases.

It also doesn't stop at only one test; further tests are done to monitor progress of the 'disease'—tests that are often expensive, invasive and stressful. According to Dr Pramod Mathur,* an endocrinologist specializing in thyroid disorders, 'A forty-three-year-old woman was referred to me by a colleague. Though all her thyroid tests were normal, my colleague had suggested a thyroid ultrasound. The ultrasound revealed a few small nodules, which the technician helpfully told her was "maybe cancer". She was a wreck when she came to me. I assured her that those nodes were normal and too minuscule, and it was highly unlikely that would be anything abnormal. I thought that I had managed to convince her and allay all her fears. After a few weeks, I saw her at another endocrinologist's waiting room.

She was highly embarrassed to see me but she said that she needed a second opinion and this doctor had prescribed medications and suggested six-monthly ultrasounds to monitor progress. Nonplussed, I challenged my colleague on his treatment plan. He pointed out that he has bills to pay and if that means telling the patient what she wants to hear, so be it. He had put her on a regimen of expensive supplements that can be purchased only from the hospital pharmacy, thus ensuring regular revenue. That's when I realized that it is not enough to be a good doctor, one needs to be a good businessman too!'

Overtreatment tends to put a heavy burden on the health system as well. Doctors are busy tending to the healthy and have little time to attend to those who are really sick. Hospital beds are occupied by people who do not really need them, leaving those who are in dire need in the lurch.

What Do We Do about It?

It is said that overdiagnosis of the well and undertreatment of the sick are 'the conjoined twins of modern medicine'.[7] Both are a reflection on the failure of the healthcare system at large. One of the major reasons for undertreatment in India is lack of access to proper medical care. Another is the issue of affordability. It is not just enough to build hospitals, we also need well-trained medical and paramedical professionals to manage them. We need strong public healthcare policies and to have equitable distribution of resources, be it infrastructure or personnel. Above all, we need to have systems in place to monitor healthcare delivery across the country. I have addressed this issue at greater length in the chapter on public health.

There are several reasons for overtreatment and overdiagnosis. The most obvious one is that unethical doctors and hospitals need to keep the cash counters busy. Also, there is patient pressure to write prescriptions and even order tests. It is a difficult task to tell a patient who needs no medication that he can go home without any prescription and will be fine. The suspicious manner in which patients view such doctors is a reason why most physicians prescribe some medication, even if it is just multivitamin tablets. Yet another reason for overtreatment is the 'why take a chance' attitude among doctors. This involves doctors knowing that a particular drug, say an antibiotic, is not indicated but going ahead with prescribing one anyway as, 'What if the patient does not improve within the next day or two and blames the doctors?'

As far as surgeries and procedures are concerned, it has been well documented that a sizable percentage of them are unnecessary. Many are performed for dubious benefits or simply to boost hospital revenues.

Another important reason for overtreatment is the plethora of studies showing 'complications' of certain diseases in a small percentage of patients several years later if left untreated. The medical community loathes to take the risk that may arise from not treating the condition for years to prevent complications. I recommend that the community adopt the theory of acceptable risk.

Everyday life is fraught with risks—car accidents, kitchen accidents, malfunctioning electrical appliances leading to death, and given the conditions of the roads in India, even walking on them is dangerous! All of us are aware of these and similar other risks, but barring a handful of really paranoid people, we continue our daily lives without living in constant terror. We have rationalized that the benefits from these actions far outweigh the risks, which anyway are miniscule in the larger context.

This is what I call the 'theory of acceptable risk'.

I believe that adoption of this theory by the medical community will definitely reduce overtreatment.

The current zero-risk tolerance approach by doctors leads to people being overtreated for a condition that could potentially be damaging, years later. It does not take into account that the vast majority of patients may not be affected at all and can continue to lead healthy lives without the complication occurring.

But who will take this decision?

Not the healthcare industry that generates millions of dollars by overtreating patients. The industry benefits from fearmongering. There is no way to definitely say who among the few will go onto develop complications after a period of time. Any government would be disinclined to take this decision that may have potential public criticism. The healthcare industry would be quick to bring this to the public's notice and use this as further proof to push treatment options.

Doctors need to find out the percentage of risk, inform the patients about it and also inform them about the risks of the treatment. Then the patient can make an informed decision. It is time that you and I take the trouble to understand the risk factors of a potential line of treatment.

Surgeons are required to explain the risks involved in any surgical procedure. There is a detailed consent form that has to be signed off by the patient or the caregiver. It is mandated that this form should be in a language that the patient understands. Any surgery would be conducted only after getting the patient's informed consent.

I believe that if this process was followed before embarking on treatment for all major or chronic conditions where the risks are known, the patient would be empowered to make an informed choice. This process can be further strengthened if the government—in consultation with independent medical professionals—publishes an officially approved annual list of known risks for specific conditions.

I am sure that there would be a surprisingly large number of patients who would seriously weigh the trade-off between quality of life and the risks, especially when the risks are small. They may benefit from taking the conservative approach rather than the additional side-effects that any treatment process will often bring.

While it may be too premature to advocate implementing such a theory into mainstream healthcare delivery in India, it may be worthwhile for health policy makers to ponder on the possibilities.

As a child, when I was taken to see my doctor, I always saw a sign that hung outside his door that read, 'I only dress the wound, God heals it.' Sadly, today, the healthcare industry is in too much of a hurry to let God heal the wounded.

To quote one of my professors, 'The best physician is one who knows when not to intervene, and the best surgeon is one who knows when not to operate.'

3

The Epidemic of Unnecessary Surgeries and Procedures

Ronojoy Ghoshal,* a schoolteacher from West Bengal, shared his experience with me: 'I took my seventy-two-year-old mother to the doctor as she complained of severe lower back pain. Since we live in a village with limited medical facilities, I took her to Kolkata to a big hospital. The hospital was huge! We met a doctor who asked some questions and advised tests. Since we were not from Kolkata, he said that it would be cheaper if we got admitted into the hospital. I could also stay in the room, and we wouldn't have to spend on hotel bookings. It seemed reasonable and we agreed. Then started a whirlwind of tests and meetings with many doctors. After a few days, they said that she needed a spinal surgery as the degeneration was too severe to be fixed with drugs. Frightened, I agreed. After spending lakhs of rupees, she was finally discharged post-surgery. When we went to the hospital, her only complaint was the lower back pain. She was fully managing her own activities in her daily life. It has been nearly a year since the surgery, and we followed all the advice of the doctor, but still, she is so weak that she can't even manage her own chores. I don't know what to do! Maybe we should have tried conservative treatment first.'

Did you know that thousands of surgeries and procedures performed every year across the world are medically unnecessary?

I am referring to the thousands of spinal fusions, joint replacements, angioplasties, C-sections, hysterectomies, etc., that are done every year—procedures that may be more beneficial to the bottom line of the hospitals than to the health of the patient.

What are the driving forces behind this epidemic? What can you, as a layperson, do to avoid being a victim of this global phenomenon?

Unnecessary Surgeries

Ankur,* a thirty-five-year-old IT executive based out of Thiruvananthapuram, shared his story with me: 'We were so thrilled when the doctor said that my wife was pregnant. Both of us were healthy and had good careers. We wanted a normal delivery, and my wife took all the necessary care. Finally, the wait was over and she went into labour. A few hours later, the doctor approached me and said that the baby was in distress and the only way to save the baby was to perform an emergency C-section. We had no choice but to agree. Much later, I found out that the doctor had done the same for three other mothers that week. Apparently, she was scheduled to go on a holiday the next day and didn't want to wait endlessly.'

Experts say that as many as one out of three surgeries (excluding cosmetic surgeries) may not be totally necessary. What are unnecessary surgeries? According to me, those procedures that: a) are not medically warranted; b) are not in the best interest of the patient; c) are undertaken before exhausting all other options are unnecessary surgeries.

> This is not a new phenomenon. As early as the 1950s, the then director of the American College of Surgeons, Dr Paul Hawley, stated that the public would be shocked if it knew the amount of unnecessary surgery that was being performed.[1] Now, this phenomenon has increased manifold. The most common unnecessary surgeries are:
>
> - Hysterectomy
> - C-sections
> - Knee and hip replacements
> - Cardiac stents
> - Pacemakers
> - Spinal surgeries
> - Gallbladder removal
> - Radical prostatectomy

There is no doubt that all these surgeries are lifesaving when medically necessary. If they're not needed, however, these surgeries often leave the patient worse off, both in terms of health and finances. Most surgeons reassure the patient by stating that these surgeries are common and routine, and that the surgeon has acquired considerable skill in the area. Still, all of this is hardly reassuring to the patient who has much more at stake—especially if there are other conservative options available!

Let us look at a few epidemics that are rampant in India.

The hysterectomy epidemic

Cheenu* was very happy when she discovered that she was pregnant. She was from a village in Telangana and was married to a carpenter, who treated her well. Unlike the horror stories she had heard of alcoholic and wife-beating husbands, her husband Jana* was a good person. They lived in a comfortable room in the city. Her pregnancy only added to their happiness. All was smooth till the delivery. She was admitted to a private hospital (her husband wanted the best for her), where the basic charges itself were quite high. As she was in labour, the doctor announced that she needed an emergency Caesarean delivery (C-section). Jana had no choice but to agree, even though the charges would be much more than he had envisaged. But that's not the end of the story. As soon as the baby was delivered, the doctors said that there was heavy bleeding and the only way to save Cheenu's life was to remove her uterus. There was no time for second opinions or even to think. Barely knowing what he had agreed to, Jana signed the consent form.

The medical expenses were around ₹1.5 lakhs, an amount they could barely afford. Jana had to take a loan to pay the bill. Today, at twenty-four, Cheenu is menopausal with myriad health issues. Faced with a never-ending cycle of debt, Jana is now an alcoholic who takes out his frustrations on his wife and child.

Unfortunately, there are thousands of Cheenus in India. The National Family Health Survey in India, 2015–16, reveals that:[2]

- Hysterectomy prevalence ranged between 3–5 per cent in 126 districts, 5–7 per cent in forty-seven districts and more than 7 per cent in twenty-six districts.
- The prevalence of hysterectomies overall was 3.2 per cent, the highest in Andhra Pradesh (8.9 per cent) and the lowest in Assam (0.9 per cent).
- Rural India had a higher prevalence of this surgery than urban India.
- The majority of women underwent the operation in private hospitals.

While hysterectomies are a common procedure and have saved the lives of millions of women across the globe, recent advances in medical science have ushered in non-surgical alternatives for some of the conditions that would have required a hysterectomy earlier. In many parts of India, however, it is still the only option that is offered to women for any menstrual problem.

A study from Andhra Pradesh[3] revealed that nearly 60 per cent of hysterectomies were conducted on women under the age of thirty—a shocking number—and 95 per cent of them were performed in private hospitals. The discharge summaries were shoddy, most of them incomplete with little or no information either on the procedure or the follow-up protocol. There is no way to find out if these women had other options than the removal of an important organ. Ironically, this increase can be attributed to the state-sponsored Rajiv Aarogyasri Health Insurance Scheme. Under this scheme, which was launched in 2007, almost 19.2 million below-poverty-line households were provided generous cashless coverage for tertiary healthcare. Private hospitals make more money under the programme by operating on more patients and billing the insurance providers directly.

The numbers eventually came down after a huge media outcry, but that offers little solace to the thousands of women who had this absolutely unnecessary procedure.

A 2011 article, 'Uterus Removal of 226 Women in Rajasthan Was a Bestial Act', revealed that four private hospitals in Rajasthan's Dausa district removed the uteruses of 226 women in 2010, earning about ₹14,000 from each patient.[4] Many of these women had gone to the hospital for health issues like stomach aches. They went to private hospitals as the government ones were not easily accessible.

Most of these women come from poor backgrounds and had to borrow money for the procedure, which trapped them in a vicious cycle of debt.

This epidemic is a clear violation of human rights. It is atrocious that a woman's reproductive rights are violated by agencies that have sworn to safeguard her health. Hysterectomies in young women can lead to multiple other problems. Even today, in many parts of India, a woman's worth is judged by her ability to bear children and barren women are often abandoned by their families.

The C-Section epidemic

'C-section or normal delivery?' This is now a common question asked when the birth of a child is announced. Caesarean delivery, or C-section, is a surgical procedure that helps deliver a baby through incisions in the mother's abdomen. It is indeed a boon when there are medical complications in labour. These complications may range from health concerns in the mother or the baby, multiple births, the baby or mother being in distress, labour not progressing, etc.

But, as the years passed, many mothers began demanding C-sections to avoid the pain associated with labour. Families wanted their heirs to be born at 'auspicious times' and planned C-sections became the norm rather than the exception, especially among those with the economic bandwidth.

But not all the C-sections are done by the patient's demands. Doctors also play an important role in persuading patients to opt for C-sections. I am given to understand that there were potentially 9 lakh preventable C-sections in the private sector in 2016.[5] That's a whopping number! Unnecessary C-sections are not just financially draining but can also cause health issues in the child. It is believed that caesarean babies are more likely to develop asthma and obesity.[6] They are also prone to transient tachypnoea of the newborn, a condition that causes rapid breathing for a few days. Other health issues can include delayed growth, respiratory morbidities and a compromised immune system. For the mother, it can mean post-labour pain, increased chances of infection, reduction in fertility and complications in future pregnancies. There is also a much higher prevalence of repeat C-sections.

An obstetrician and gynaecologist (Ob/gyn), Dr Sapna Vaidya* provides more context: 'I have my own hospital in a small town. I am the only Ob/gyn in the hospital. My days are packed with regular patients, and I need to be at my clinic most of the day. I am also a mother and have to tend to my family. A normal delivery can go on for hours. On an average, I have seven to ten patients a week in labour. Imagine the number of hours I would have to spend if each of them opts for normal delivery! I may as well forget about eating and sleeping. So, I gently coax a few of the mothers to opt for a C-section, even if they are not medically necessary. But unlike a few of my colleagues, who blindly perform C-sections, I try to identify those patients who have the capacity to pay. After all, a C-section can be three to four times as expensive as a normal delivery.' Honour among thieves, indeed! But Dr Vaidya has a point: not all doctors and hospitals bother about the financial capabilities of the patient. As I have mentioned multiple times, patients across the country are increasingly opting for private medical facilities as there is not much faith in government medical services. The private medical industry is highly unregulated and has largely escaped accountability, though of late there have been certain changes. As long as there is a financial incentive for generating additional revenue for the hospital, women across the country will be subjected to unnecessary C-sections.

The stent epidemic

The last few decades have seen an increase in cardiovascular diseases among Indians. Genetic predisposition, lifestyle changes, unhealthy dietary choices, increasing stress levels have all contributed to this. Unsurprisingly, there is a parallel increase in surgical interventions to arrest these diseases. Angioplasty and stent placement are common procedures that help in opening up clogged arteries in the heart. The process involves the use of a tiny balloon to widen the artery and the inserting of a tiny wire-mesh tube to prevent the artery from closing. In medical terminology, these procedures are known as coronary angioplasty, or percutaneous coronary intervention (PCI). Typically, these procedures are recommended for acute heart problems—in other words, for heart attacks or pre-heart attack symptoms. A report by the National Interventional Council of Cardiological Society of India (CSI–NIC)[7] reveals that in

2018, a total of 5,78,164 stents were used, out of which 98.12 per cent were drug-eluting stents (DES). A DES is coated with slow-release medication that helps prevent plaque buildup in the arteries.

How many of these procedures were really necessary? It is indeed difficult to estimate the number as there are no regulations in place to capture the essential data. Studies conducted in the US, where there is more robust data collection, revealed that only 50 per cent of non-emergency cardiac stenting were medically necessary.[8] Further investigation showed a nexus of kickbacks between a few stent manufacturers and doctors. If that was the case in a highly regulated environment like the US, what do you think will be the scenario in India, with no audit or regulation in place? This concern is endorsed by the eminent cardiac surgeon Dr Devi Shetty, chairman of Narayana Health:[9] 'I agree that a significant percentage of angioplasties are inappropriate. I think that the Cardiology Society of India should bring out guidelines and create a mechanism to audit themselves rather than giving a chance for an external body to be created. Such an audit is needed as society has lost trust in doctors because of such inappropriate use (of stents).'

Historically, stents have been major money spinners for hospitals. Till 2017, hospitals were not required to give the details of the brand of stents used or their price in the final bill presented to the patient. This meant that the patient could end up paying a higher charge for a lower cost stent. Hospitals would make a profit margin as high as 650 per cent in some cases!

Finally, in 2017, the National Pharmaceutical Pricing Authority (NPPA)[10] made a landmark announcement decreeing that hospitals must list out all details—including the brand name, lot number, price, etc., of the stents. This brought in much needed relief to the patient.

Ronika Mishra,* a college professor from Lucknow, recalls, 'My father was advised to get a stent and we admitted him to a leading hospital in Mumbai. We were told that the cost of the procedure can be anything to the tune of ₹2 lakh to ₹2.5 lakh. We did not have insurance and we struggled to raise the money. We somehow managed it, and my father was taken in for the surgery. As we waited anxiously, one of the attending doctors came from inside the OT and informed us that there are more blocks than what were earlier seen, and additional stents would be needed. The additional expenses? Two lakhs more. We had to save our father and we agreed to the procedure. It was only much later, when we spoke to a few other people, that we realized this was a common modus operandi at that hospital. Many of them ended up paying much more than what was the initial amount for the extra stents. As laypeople, we have no resources to check the veracity of the information. And how do we get a second opinion when my father is in the OT, in the middle of a procedure? I do not have enough proof or the financial resources to take the hospital to court. But all my instincts scream that if there are so many similar cases, it needs to be investigated. As a family, we are still paying off the debts and my father blames himself for our financial condition. Me—I blame the hospital and their greed.'

Renowned cardiologist and former vice chancellor of Manipal University, Dr B.M. Hegde opines that angioplasty has a proven track record only in specific situations.[11] Otherwise, he says that it is more of a money-making tool which works by instilling fear in the patients.

One of the cardiologists we spoke to said on the strict condition of anonymity, 'I agree that at least 20–25 per cent of stenting I do are medically unnecessary. But it is a Catch-22 situation. Most of my patients are busy executives, who claim that they cannot make lifestyle changes. They have unhealthy diets, disturbed sleep patterns and high levels of stress. Many of them are heavy smokers and/or drinkers. A few of them do try to change their lifestyle, but sooner or later, fall off the bandwagon. It is easier to spend a few hours in the operation theatre than many futile hours counselling them. And it doesn't hurt that I make lakhs if I operate and only a few thousands if I counsel!'

The knee replacement epidemic

Chronic knee pain is debilitating. It affects the quality of life and confines many to an unproductive life. For such patients, a knee replacement is nothing short of a miracle. This is a process in which the diseased knee joint is removed and replaced with an artificial one. A total knee replacement (TKR) is recommended if the patient has severe arthritis (rheumatoid arthritis, osteoarthritis or any other arthritis that affects the knee) or a severe knee injury which has damaged cartilage. The surgery is advised for those patients who are in severe pain, even when resting, and whose movements are severely restricted due to pain.

Even a decade ago, this procedure was not as common as it is today. But with increased obesity and incidence of arthritis among Indians, the rates of this surgery are rising across the country.

Are these surgeries really essential? Over the last few years, newer methods like stem cell or platelet rich plasma injections into the joint have also emerged, which are far less expensive and have shown promising results. These methods are also less invasive and hence do not cause as much harm as surgeries.

In an interview with Mrs Rati More,* a sixty-eight-year-old homemaker from Navsari, Gujarat, says, 'I started developing knee pain when I was around fifty-five. The doctors gave me some medicines and asked me to lose weight. As if that is easy! Anyway, as the years passed, the pain increased, and my son took me to a big specialist in Delhi. That doctor just saw me for ten minutes and advised a knee surgery. We didn't know much about it but I would have done anything to become better. The whole procedure, including the surgery, our trips to Delhi, stay, etc., cost us around ₹5 lakhs. After the surgery, there was a lot of physiotherapy, and it took me more than three months to walk around freely. But slowly, the pain came back and now the doctors are saying that the problem was not in my knee but that it was referred pain from the hip and there was perhaps no need for the knee replacement at all! Now, they are suggesting hip replacement. How do I trust them?

Do I just have to accept that I will be in pain for the rest of my life and that I cannot move around much or replace yet another joint in the hope of getting well?'

One of the surgeons we spoke to, on the grounds of anonymity, said, 'I agree that many a time, we do surgeries that are not really warranted. I was headhunted by this major chain of corporate hospital and my name is used in all their advertisements. I am responsible for bringing in a certain amount of revenue every year. How can I meet this target if I counsel patients to modify their lifestyle, go to a physiotherapist, etc.? Anyway, I know that most of them won't have the discipline to follow a routine. And they will go around saying that they came to me and I didn't help them and that I am not a good doctor. And then they will go to someone else, who will perform the surgery. It is easier for me to do a knee replacement. The patient feels that I have done something, the hospital earns revenue and my reputation is intact. I know that some of my colleagues snidely refer to me as the king of knee replacements but I prefer to take it as a compliment!'

To quote the UAE-based consultant rheumatologist and my good friend, Dr Humeira Badsha, 'Surgeries are not recommended for everyone. It is advisable only when the cartilage or joints are highly damaged and the patient has high levels of pain, affecting their quality of life. I often see X-rays where the knees are highly damaged with significant loss of cartilage, but the patient is functional and can go about their daily activities with minimal pain. I would encourage these patients to consult a qualified physiotherapist and follow the prescribed exercise regimen. Surgery is always the last resort, only after all other options have been exhausted.'

Are the surgeons listening?

Why Do Surgeons Perform Unnecessary Surgeries?

From the beginning of organized medicine, doctors have been urged to consider the patient's welfare above all. 'Do no harm' is the mantra for all doctors. How did this change? Why are we seeing an upswing in unnecessary surgeries? Is it just greed or are there any other reasons?

Patient's insistence

Dr Sameer Sheikh,* a Bhopal-based surgeon, shares his experience: 'The other day I had a patient who came in with severe knee pain. He was a local politician with a lot of clout in the area. After studying his various reports and clinically examining him, I recommended physiotherapy and that he loses weight. He was not happy with my opinion. He said that he knew of people who became better after a knee surgery and that is what he needed. His entourage also echoed the same sentiments. They insisted that I perform the surgery. Though it went against the very essence of what I believe, I had to perform the surgery. Obviously, he had some relief after the post-surgery recovery period. But I know that he can develop symptoms again. I dread to think of what my situation would be when that happens!'

With 'Dr Google', every patient—especially the urban, educated population—is a medical 'expert'. Many of them have busy lives and cannot—or more accurately, do not—make time for exercising and lifestyle changes. For them, a surgical option seems to be the easier choice. Physiotherapist Mark Lobo* shares, 'It is not just that it is an easier choice. Sometimes, patients are in so much pain that they will do anything to have a better quality of life. While physiotherapy and lifestyle changes can help, they cannot always cure, say, an arthritis patient. It is not easy to live a compromised life, so many people think that if there is even a 50 per cent chance of getting a better life with surgery, why not give that a go?' Additionally, patients are often, not fully informed about the risks of the surgery and that not all patients undergoing it will do well after the procedure.

Not considering choices

To practise medicine, one has to be a lifelong learner. What I learned as a medical student may not necessarily be the optimal protocol today. There are much better pharmacological approaches available now, than a decade ago. Physiotherapy is another area that has advanced by leaps and bounds. The fifty-two-year-old HR executive Mahika Pant recalls,* 'I was diagnosed with rheumatoid arthritis [R.A.] in 1998. It was a tough time for me. The pain was unbearable, and I was barely functional. There was no rheumatologist in the small town I lived in, and I was seeing an orthopaedist. By 2005, my knee pain was unbearable, and he recommended surgery as the only option. My cousin, who lived in the US, was also diagnosed with R.A. around the same time and she insisted that I consult with her doctor for a second opinion. I travelled to the US and met with her rheumatologist, who changed my medications and advised physiotherapy. It was very difficult in the beginning, but within a few months, there was a dramatic improvement in my pain levels and my movement. If my cousin hadn't intervened, I would have had the surgery that may not have really helped.'

Multiple research papers[12] in the past few years have revealed that physiotherapy helps in the early stages of certain musculoskeletal problems. It delays further deterioration and can prevent surgical intervention. These research papers also reveal that, in certain cases, the long-term effects of physiotherapy and surgery are the same. According to physiotherapist Suchi Diwakar,* 'Many patients feel that physiotherapy is a long-drawn process. They want quick results. Also, they need to put in all the hard work. We can only guide them, but they need to make the changes and stick to the recommended exercise protocol. They feel that it is easier to go under the knife. What they don't understand is that for complete recovery, a post-surgery rehabilitation programme is a must. Isn't it better then to try out the non-surgical option first? After all, exercise helps in multiple ways!'

Are patients and doctors listening?

Targets and corporate greed

As I have mentioned multiple times in the book, greed is the biggest motivator. Investors are eager to make more money and consider the healthcare industry as a money-making enterprise rather than an altruistic one. Unrealistic targets, unethical practices, market economics, competition—all these factors play an important role as well.

To Cut or Not to Cut?

Being a physician is tough, being a surgeon is tougher. It requires a special kind of skill and mental aptitude to become a surgeon. It is also one of the most rewarding professions in the world. And with this comes the responsibility of always putting the interests of the patient first. This means that surgeons must take a stand against unnecessary surgeries that put the patient at risk. A patient-centric approach is the need of the hour.

There needs to be stringent guidelines to protect the patient's interests. There has been considerable progress on this front with the capping of prices of stents and artificial joints. But that is not enough. Whether it is a hysterectomy or a hip transplant, no surgery should be performed unless it is medically necessary and only after all the other options have been exhausted. For now, though, the epidemic of unnecessary surgeries seems set to continue.

4
Is the Quality of Healthcare Being Measured?

In my early years of medical practice, I worked in a paediatric intensive care unit as a registrar. One of my patients was a child of around nine or ten years old, who was admitted with polyneuropathy, or Guillain-Barré Syndrome. The child was paralysed. He was on a ventilator and connected to an endotracheal tube and a feeding tube. His health showed signs of improvement and we were progressively weaning him off the ventilator. One morning, at around 5.30 a.m., I rushed to the hospital following a call informing me that the child had developed sudden respiratory distress and his vitals were unstable. On examination, I found that fluid had entered his lungs. I was told that he was fed a few minutes before he went into distress. Closer examination revealed a few drops of milk in the endotracheal tube. By mistake, a nurse had likely pushed some milk into the endotracheal tube instead of the nasogastric tube or maybe the child aspirated as he was being fed.

The child did not survive. This is an extreme example, but this episode left a major impact on me. We had developed a bond with the child, and he had been showing signs of recovery. We had been hopeful of getting him out of the ICU by the end of that week.

There was an inquiry that revealed nothing as the nurses denied any role in the fiasco. The hospital management also thought that it was prudent to gloss over the incident, like many others. Even if there is significant evidence of something that has gone wrong, nothing is really done by the management to prevent a recurrence. And these are hospitals that pride themselves on the quality of their healthcare services!

What cannot be measured cannot be improved. Nowhere is this adage truer than in healthcare. In an area where precision is a matter of life and death, it is imperative that we measure the quality-of-care delivery to the maximum extent possible. Some areas of quality measurement are relatively straightforward.

For example, questions like the following can be answered and measured easily:

- Were treatment protocols followed within expected timelines?
- Were checklists complied with?
- What were the outcomes of procedures, surgeries and non-invasive treatments?

Some others are more difficult to measure, like patient satisfaction indices, soft skills of doctors and staff, etc.

The government itself does not measure many quality indices in its institutions. The few that it measures are easy to fudge. Obviously, then, the quality of healthcare delivery in India is more or less unknown. While there is indirect evidence from, say, reduction in infectious diseases in an area, fall in infant and maternal mortality rates, etc., by and large we have no idea at all about the quality of care that an individual hospital or doctor provides.

Whether easy or difficult, there is no doubt of the burning need to measure the quality of healthcare delivery on an ongoing basis. Unfortunately, there is virtually no significant system in place in India for this.

Some corporate hospitals do measure a few indices but they are mostly limited to the area of patient satisfaction and not in the core domain of healthcare delivery. This, too, is usually done with an eye on revenues.

There is no compulsion from the government to measure quality, so private hospitals have no reason to measure the quality of their services. An even more significant reason is that hospitals themselves fear what might emerge if this Pandora's box is opened.

Questions such as how many patients who underwent a surgical procedure in a particular hospital or with a particular surgeon recovered, how many succumbed, how many had complications, etc.—are at best a guesstimate. There is no record even of infection rates in hospital ICUs, the number of adverse drug reactions, cases where wrong dosages of drugs were prescribed, etc. You could be at the plushest hospital with seven-star facilities, but it is probable that no one is actually measuring any of the vital data that could potentially be lifesaving. This is where we are today. No one—neither the government, healthcare industry, pharmaceutical companies nor the diagnostics industry—no one is really working to change it.

There are a few committed and motivated doctors who do measure critical data. Their motivations are the pride they derive from their work and their commitment to excellence rather than any material compulsion.

What People Say

The other day, I was chatting with a friend who migrated to the US decades ago. Like many others in the throes of the first COVID-19 wave, we were using the lockdown to connect with long-lost friends. As we chatted, I asked her if she missed Chennai at all. She replied, 'You have no idea how much I miss it! It is the city where I grew up, where my friends are—it is home to me, even after twenty-five years of life in the US. I frequently think about returning to India. But the biggest hurdle as we grow older is the quality of healthcare. You know that with my health condition, I need frequent hospital visits and doctor consults. While the quality of doctors and medical expertise in India is world-class, what is lacking is the quality of care. I do not know if the hospital staff have followed all protocols and procedures. Also, the little things that make hospital visits bearable—the soft qualities like empathy, compassion, communication, maybe?' While the patriot in me wanted to furiously argue, I had to agree with her point. Quality of care is the least important factor in most Indian hospitals. How often have we gone to the 'best' of hospitals and left fuming at the quality of care?

Thirty-seven-year-old data analyst Mithun Saha* recounts his experience: 'My father had just undergone a prostrate removal surgery and he was super cranky. He kept asking to see the doctor wanted to clarify some doubts. Instead of answering his questions, the nurse on duty was rude to him and said that he is old enough to take a little discomfort, which would anyway be there. Contrast this with my friend's experience in the US. The doctors took the time to explain the procedure at length before the actual surgery. After the procedure, the surgeon visited him and answered all his questions patiently, even though he had addressed all his concerns earlier. I understand that the staff are overworked in India, but is a little kindness too much to ask for?'

This is a story that proves that there are doctors who see patients as humans and not just cases. We spoke to forty-three-year-old journalist Meghana Rudra,* who said, 'My teenage daughter complained of intense stomach pain, and we rushed her to the emergency room. After observation and some diagnostics, they said that the appendix needs to be removed and the surgery was scheduled for the day after. Her pain was under control and she was comfortable. But she had one issue. She had been selected as a prefect in her school and the investiture ceremony was the next morning.

She was complaining about missing it and bemoaning her fate when the doctor came on his rounds. He asked why she was sad and, after hearing her out, he said that since there was no immediate threat to her health, she can be given a temporary discharge for two hours—just to attend the ceremony and receive her prefect's badge. He didn't have to do this but this small gesture made her so happy! It also helped in allaying her fears of the surgery as "Doctor Uncle" was now her hero!'

'My grandmother was admitted to the ICU of a leading corporate hospital for what was suspected to be a rhythm abnormality of the heart. She was recovering but twenty-four hours later, when I went to see her, she was restless and shouting, repeatedly asking for water. We started wondering about her state of mind when we found that she had received neither IV fluids nor anything by mouth for the entire duration of the previous day, since the time of admission. IV fluids had been suggested by the doctor in the emergency department but another doctor in the ICU had suggested oral feeding. In the confusion, the patient got neither. And the charges for treatment in that ICU? As high as ₹1 lakh per day,' rants twenty-nine-year-old PhD scholar Tamanna Grover.*

A lot of this has to do with the basics. Think of a time you visited a doctor in the pre-COVID days in India. It may have been for some common flu-like symptoms. The doctor may have examined you and arrived at some diagnosis. After their examination, did they wash their hands? And think of changing the sheet on the examination table. I know that many doctors still use cloth sheets, and these are not changed between patients. Even during the peak of the pandemic, a friend had a similar experience. She says, 'I had to go in for an abdominal ultrasound. Though it was during the pandemic, I could not avoid it and booked an appointment at what was touted to be the best diagnostic centre in the city. I had to travel quite far but thought it was preferable in those days. Imagine my horror when I saw little social distancing being maintained in the waiting area. There was no sanitizer dispenser in the room. I was called into the scan room as the previous patient was leaving and no one changed the sheets! Furious, I asked for the manager to lodge a complaint. When I was ushered into his cabin, he was sitting there not wearing a mask! I just walked out of the centre.'

This was a diagnostic centre in a posh area of Hyderabad, not some backwoods village. A lab may have the best equipment, technician and doctor on their rolls, but is that enough to ensure quality of care?

Every year, preventable infections, mostly diarrhoeal diseases and pneumonia, kill hundreds of thousands of Indians, especially children, in hospitals that range from the dirty, desperately staffed government facilities to the plush corporate hospitals of our metros. Every year, worldwide, 30,000 women and 4 lakh babies die from infections such as puerperal sepsis, often caused by lack of water, sanitation and poor handwashing practices.[1] It is estimated that 22 lakh children under the age of five die each year due to diarrhoeal diseases and pneumonia alone, with the vast majority of deaths occurring in just five countries. At least 25 per cent of these deaths could potentially be prevented just by the attending medical team washing their hands with soap. The Centers for Disease Control and Prevention in the US runs an annual full-fledged campaign titled 'Clean Hands Save lives'. Every year, 15 October is observed as Global Handwashing Day around the world. Yet, precious little is done in India to ensure that even simple aseptic precautions are taken. The WHO estimates that among children under the age of five in India, 3.7 lakh die from pneumonia and 3.34 lakh die from diarrhoea each year. That's a whopping 7.04 lakh children under five years of age! With good hygiene alone, at least one-fourth of them can be saved—that's almost 1.76 lakh children each year. Did we need a pandemic to force us to adopt a lifesaving habit? Did we have a sustained campaign promoting handwashing? Did our hospitals insist that the correct aseptic precautions be followed? The answer to all these questions is a big fat 'No.'

Why? Simple! Where is the money? You cannot fatten your wallet by promoting this simple yet effective routine. Of course, the soap companies can, and they are doing their bit, but what about the healthcare industry?

What EXACTLY Is Quality of Care?

Quality of care is the degree to which health services for individuals and populations increase the likelihood of desired health outcomes and are consistent with evidence-based professional knowledge.

Let us dissect this definition, which shall lead to many questions: how can one ensure an increase in the desired health outcomes? While treatment is important, isn't it more important to prevent incidence of diseases? And isn't post-treatment rehabilitation critical to ensure a healthy population? What about education on how to prevent and manage health conditions? How important are cultural and socio-economic factors in providing healthcare? What about the needs and preferences of service users—patients, families and communities?

Obviously, there are many elements to quality. The WHO decrees quality health services should be:[2]

- effective by providing evidence-based healthcare services to those who need them.
- safe by avoiding harm to the people for whom the care is intended.
- people-centred by providing care that responds to individual preferences, needs and values within health services that are organized around the needs of people.
- timely by reducing waiting times and sometimes harmful delays for both those who receive and those who give care.
- equitable by providing the same quality of care regardless of age, sex, gender, race, ethnicity,

geographic location, religion, socio-economic status, linguistic or political affiliation.

- integrated by providing care that is coordinated across levels and providers and makes available the full range of health services throughout the course of life.
- efficient by maximizing the benefit of available resources and avoiding waste.

Quality of care is closely intertwined with ethical principles and practices. The healthcare industry cannot delink these two factors and expect to serve the larger population. In India, it is correct to say that very little is being measured. Again, among what is being measured, the bulk of it is quantitative. Quality indicators are slowly being introduced, but the data is very limited as there is no compulsion to keep track of it.

The general attitude amongst the powers that be is that as long as they are not legally mandated to measure quality of care, why bother at all?

Different Perceptions of Quality

It is interesting to note that there is not a single universally accepted definition of quality as a concept. In many ways, it can be subjective. Healthcare quality is even more complex to measure, given the wide range of services, the unique needs of each patient or the population, the laws of the land, etc. A hospital may offer high-quality infrastructure but a doctor there may have limited knowledge or poor bedside manner. Or the doctor may be excellent but the nurse assigned to you may be apathetic. Or all the services may be excellent but the patient may have come in a little too late or have an incurable condition and may succumb to the disease. There are so many variables that can go right or wrong.

On the other hand, if you were buying a car, you have adequate measurable parameters to arrive at a measure of quality. An automobile manufacturer can churn out consistent quality. But the same cannot be said of a healthcare provider. The same disease does not affect all patients in exactly the same way. The COVID-19 pandemic has proven this over and over again. I have seen an eighty-five-year-old with comorbidities have a largely mild attack while, at the same time, a twenty-eight-year-old with no previous health complaints succumb to the disease. In either case, the healthcare offered to them did not affect the outcome. The attending medical team was the same and they rigorously followed all the recommended protocols in both cases. In such situations, we then resort to the old lament 'It was fate! Who can do anything about this?'

The perception of quality also varies depending on who the stakeholder is.

For the patient, a clean hospital with polite, receptive and communicative doctors and staff signifies quality (as long as they recover).

To a surgeon, a clean procedure with minimal blood loss, a healthy wound and no postoperative infection could signify quality.

For a hospital administrator, on-time availability of infrastructure and resources leading to their optimum utilization may denote quality.

In essence, all these taken together form a part of the quality construct. It is just that some are more important than others to individual stakeholders, depending on which side of the fence they are on.

A patient does not know the difference between minimal and moderate blood loss, or a minimal scar versus a slightly larger one. They would not know if clinical protocols were observed strictly or if infection control methods were adopted, etc.

Likewise, the surgeon has no idea whether the billing manager was communicative or rude, or whether the cleanliness in the room was maintained at all times and so on.

While quality is a matter of perception depending on many factors, it can also be subjective. What may be acceptable to me may not be acceptable to you. But it is an extremely critical factor in healthcare and one that needs to be measured by all healthcare providers. Let's take a quick look at some data on the current quality of health services, as determined by the WHO:[3]

- Between 5.7 and 8.4 million deaths are attributed to poor quality care each year in low- and middle-income countries (LMICs), which represents up to 15 per cent of overall deaths in these countries.

- Sixty per cent of deaths in LMICs from conditions requiring healthcare occur due to poor quality care, whereas the remaining deaths result from non-utilization of the health system.

- Inadequate quality of care imposes costs of US $1.4–1.6 trillion each year in lost productivity in LMICs.

- In high-income countries, one in ten patients is harmed while receiving hospital care, and seven in every 100 hospitalized patients can expect to acquire a healthcare-associated infection.

- It has been estimated that high quality health systems could prevent 2.5 million deaths from cardiovascular disease, 900,000 deaths from tuberculosis, 1 million newborn deaths and half of all maternal deaths each year.

- Globally, the essential structures for achieving quality care are inadequate: one in eight healthcare facilities has no water service, one in five has no sanitation service, and one in six has no hand hygiene facilities at the points of care.

- An estimated 1.8 billion people, or 24 per cent of the world's population, live in fragile contexts that are challenged in delivering quality essential health services. A large proportion of preventable maternal, childhood and neonatal deaths occur in these settings.

Hence, we need to look at the quality of healthcare from a holistic perspective to ensure we are measuring all the important parameters.

What Factors Influence Quality of Care?

There are many factors that influence the quality of care. What is acceptable quality for a person who lives in the remote villages of India may not be so for an Indian who has lived in a developed Western country for decades. It also depends on the interpersonal relationships between the doctor and the patients. It is not uncommon to find two members of the same family having completely opposing views on the care provided by the same physician.

Social factors play a big role in defining the quality of care. I remember an incident where a panchayat chief was furious that a female doctor was appointed as the chief of the local government clinic. It did not comply with the village's existing patriarchal society. I also know of a very wealthy and ultra conservative family in Mumbai who refused to consult a male doctor for any of the female members of the family. There was this one time when one of the women in the family suffered a hip fracture. Instead of taking her to the nearest orthopaedic facility, the family was searching for a facility with a female orthopaedist.

In a country like India, language plays an important role in measuring the quality of care too. Even if the language is the same, the variation in dialects makes it impossible for us to understand patients sometimes. Critical information often gets lost in translation.

Education levels and the socio-economic status tend to affect quality. According to Dr Sudipto Banerjee,* a GP from Jharkhand, 'When a patient comes to see me, their expectation is that I will cure them by prescribing medications. However, not all cases justify this route. In many cases, what the patient needs is a protocol that consists of rest, food and exercise. I spend more time counselling patients than prescribing medications. But this approach is easier with the younger, educated lot. With others, it is like talking to a wall!'

Is it a wonder then that many doctors find it much easier to write out a prescription with a few drugs than to counsel the patient?

Educated patients are also generally more aware of their rights and, hence, more demanding when it comes to quality of care.

Leadership plays a critical role in the quality of care being offered by the hospital. If the hospital management does not provide clear metrics for monitoring and improving quality of care, how will this value permeate through all the employees in the hospital? More often than not, the leadership is rarely held accountable for quality transgressions, even if it happens on their watch. Isn't it their responsibility to establish and implement best quality practices? Isn't it their role to invest in the best of technology? What about creating a quality-oriented workplace culture? These cannot be left to the whims of individuals. Rather, a collective will would be required to create a culture of quality.

But how does one measure quality? It is, after all, an abstract concept and one that is highly subjective. But, over the years, we have defined quality parameters for almost all industries. Why should healthcare be any different? One of the popular models of our times to measure quality care is the Donabedian model.[4] It suggests that there are three fundamental elements to define quality: structure, process and outcomes.

To further simplify the model, it urges the professional to consider these questions:

- How is care organized? What is the context in which it occurs?
- What is done during the interaction with the patient?
- What is the end result of the interaction? What happens to the health of the patient?

Answering these questions will help measure quality of care. A lapse in any one of these steps will affect the final quality of care and the health of the patient.

All these factors are measurable.

The first question of structure can be measured on the basis of number of beds available per unit of population, number of doctors and nursing care per unit of population, availability of critical care facilities, availability of medical equipment, etc.

The second question is about the process. How long did the patient have to wait? Did the attending doctor or nurse make them feel comfortable? Did the patient feel heard? This data can be captured by observing consultations, feedback from patients and families and appropriate medical records.

Outcome can be measured by the number of deaths and recoveries, cost of recoveries, incidence of complications, etc.

Thanks to technology, measuring aspects of care is now easier. But the practice is largely limited to developed countries and is still difficult in the Indian scenario, where data capturing is still at a very nascent stage in most hospitals.

'My father was having some blood-pressure fluctuations and his doctor advised him to use a twenty-four-hour BP monitor. This doctor had his own clinic. He said that the monitor would be available at one of the city's big corporate hospitals. I called the hospital and was given an appointment. The traffic situation in our city is terrible and it took us almost ninety minutes to get to the hospital. After waiting for an hour, despite arriving on time for the appointment, we were told that they had run out of monitors and asked us to go to another branch, which was at the opposite end of the city—and to hurry, as they would close soon. Imagine dragging an eighty-five-year-old man from one end of the city to the other! He was exhausted by the time we returned home and refused to have anything to do with the monitor, hospitals or doctors. He claimed that he deserved to live the rest of his life in peace. It was a nightmare!' says Anitha Shetty,* a finance professional.

Anitha's experience is not unique. In her case, it was not an immediate life-and-death situation. But how many lives are lost because of the 'available on paper but unavailable in reality' facilities?

'World-class facilities', 'best of best medical staff', 'top-class equipment'—these are just a few of the terms that pepper press releases and advertisements of healthcare facilities. Alas, there is many a slip between the proverbial cup and the lip!

Most hospitals lay out stringent quality measurement guidelines for infrastructure, availability of equipment, qualification of medical staff, availability of beds per patient, etc. But much of what is listed on the quality measurement checklist are mechanically ticked off during management review and then life goes on.

I know of hospitals that have invested in quality medical equipment. But patients in the area need not necessarily have timely access to it. Even a cursory look at many hospitals, both private and government, in the country will show the real picture: equipment that is not serviced regularly, power outages affecting the functioning of the equipment, ambient temperature required for some equipment not maintained—the list of issues is endless.

A hospital may have an in-house pharmacy. That ticks the infrastructure quality checkbox. But does the pharmacy stock generic drugs? Is the cost parameter being measured?

The hospital may have top-notch doctors. But how much do the doctors know about their patients? In the words of Dr Vivek Arora,* a Kolkata-based general surgeon, 'There is no patient-information system in place. I have no idea about their medical history, current medications, etc. Not all patients maintain medical records or even remember their medications. I am often told, "I take some white pill for something for my heart, and one long pill for something." How do I treat the patient based on this information? Ask them to return with all the relevant details? Just wing it and leave the rest to a higher power?'

The irony is that despite his personal misgivings, he is rated as one of the top doctors in the hospital and always scores high on patient feedback.

How to Ensure Quality of Care in India

A 2018 study on mortality due to low-quality health systems reveals that almost 122 Indians per lakh die due to poor quality of care each year.[4] This means that India's death rate due to poor care quality is worse than that of Brazil (74), Russia (91), China (46) and South Africa (93), and even its neighbours Pakistan (119), Nepal (93), Bangladesh (57) and Sri Lanka (51).

While many of the challenges are not unique to India, it is a shame that even after decades of Independence, we still are woefully underequipped when it comes to healthcare delivery.

Here are a few hard truths:[5]

- Ninety-five per cent of healthcare facilities in India function with less than five workers.
- Only 817 (from over approximately 60,000) hospitals in the country operate with quality certifications.
- Essential diagnostics such as mammograms have a scant 1 per cent coverage across India.
- Healthcare professionals in rural areas with requisite formal medical training do not provide significantly higher-quality care when compared to informal providers or quacks.
- Private sector care does not necessarily translate to better quality of care.
- Lack of universal health coverage, access and affordability across the country remains a major challenge.

The National Accreditation Board for Hospitals & Healthcare Providers (NABH) was set up in 2005 to establish and operate accreditation programmes for healthcare providers in the country. The board has done some good work in this area. However, it is not mandatory for all hospitals to get certified, and the reach of the board is largely limited to hospital networks in bigger cities and towns. What about the tens of thousands of nursing homes that haven't bothered with NABH and blatantly violate regulations? What about the NABH-certified hospitals, who do the same?

Again, the indices they put together are more related to infrastructure and are focused on the ability of the hospital to deliver care. There is no daily mechanism in place to monitor if the accredited hospitals and labs are adhering to defined protocols. A periodic inspection does little more than provide a snapshot of their infrastructure and staffing patterns, and is a far cry from being able to reliably measure care. The net result is that hospitals and labs now boast of NABH certification to tell clients that they adhere to quality standards, while all that the certification does is to assess if they *could* deliver quality care, not if they actually *do*.

The government has, over the years, introduced many interventions to promote quality promotions: the Indian Public Health Standards 2008, National Quality Assurance Standards (NQAS) 2013, Mera-Aspataal (My Hospital) 2016, Labour Room Quality Improvement Initiative (LaQshya) 2017, and National Patient Safety Implementation Framework (2018–25).

But what is missing is a national body for monitoring quality of healthcare delivery. Organizations like the Agency for Healthcare Research and Quality (AHQR) in the US and the Care Quality Commission (CQC) in the UK monitor nationwide healthcare delivery and ensure that quality care is delivered to patients.

Shouldn't the government set up a national monitoring agency that will regularly and impartially monitor clinical quality and make this data available to the public? If this is done, hospitals will be forced to establish, maintain and monitor good clinical practices. The carrot-and-stick approach of rewarding facilities that consistently deliver high standards of care and penalizing defaulters will also help build a quality-conscious system.

Take other countries, for example. In the US, the AHRQ not only monitors quality but also introduces measures to improve it. Using one such intervention, the Comprehensive Unit-based Safety Program (CUSP),[6] Detroit-based Henry Ford Hospital reduced the percentage of central line-associated bloodstream infections (CLABSIs) in its haematology-oncology unit by 75 per cent. This reduction not only helped patients, but also saved an estimated $385,000.

Successive central and state governments have pumped crores of rupees into building infrastructure. But is that the only solution? Is the healthcare delivery system equitable? Do all Indians have equal access to quality healthcare? How long will we accept economic disparities, geographic inequities and social distinctions?

India is one among a large number of countries, mostly in the developing world, that focuses predominantly on quantitative healthcare. This means that governments believe deploying large numbers of doctors, nurses, medical equipment and hospitals will ensure quality healthcare delivery. Hence, the focus is on opening more medical and nursing colleges, building more hospitals and procuring more of the latest medical equipment. Coincidentally, the public also views the creation of these assets not just as quantitative delivery but as signs of quality as well.

A doctor missing a diagnosis or giving the wrong medication to a patient will hardly be noticed at a village healthcare centre as people will simply not know any better. But the absence of a doctor for a week could lead to a riot. The focus on getting a person in a white coat in front of the patient often subsumes everything else in healthcare delivery.

Doctor has seen patient = healthcare goals achieved.

We continue to mechanically measure indices like Infant Mortality Rate (IMR), Maternal Mortality Rate (MMR), etc., and set targets without even analysing if the improvement in those indices occurred because of our interventions or due to other factors. For example, reduction in IMR and MMR may largely be due to the arrival of better antibiotics or greater awareness among the community, rather than the larger number of hospital beds provided in villages.

Quality in healthcare is difficult to measure. Governments find it more problematic because it could reveal lacunae in their healthcare system. And since the average patient really does not know about the quality anyway (beyond general cleanliness of the hospital, etc.), many governments have neither the inclination nor the will to put in systems to measure the quality of the care delivered.

Make no mistake, quantitative healthcare is very important too. Without the expertise, equipment and infrastructure, it would be nearly impossible to deliver quality care. But what quantitative healthcare measures tell us is the *capacity* or *ability* to deliver quality care and a broad high-level view on outcomes, not whether quality care is actually being delivered at the individual level.

In the private sector, quality indices are often a hinderance, exposing dangerous shortcomings that need expensive solutions, and therefore need to be papered over as no hospital wants to spend a rupee more than absolutely necessary. Solutions may involve adding staff or equipment or even designating specific areas for certain activities, none of which add to the revenue of the hospital directly. Where then is the incentive to invest in such measures?

Why go through the headache of measuring the quality indicators and finding out that you are well short of providing quality healthcare when you are unwilling to fix it anyway? That is the attitude of most of the private sector in India.

Take, for example, outcome assessment. Hospitals have little idea of how many patients, who underwent a particular surgery or procedure, recovered without any complications. There are of course individual doctors and hospitals who do follow these numbers out of their own interest, but in most cases the hospital has no idea about the success rates of their surgeons and other doctors. Indeed, they know very little about their doctors beyond the revenues generated by them. Do hospitals know if their top surgeon has had several preventable disasters recently? They may know this through the nurses or junior doctors' whisper network, but not through a formal mechanism for identifying the same. In a country like India, 'lost to follow-up' is an easy excuse for not measuring outcomes. However, that same excuse does not prevent the hospital from sending SMS reminders to patients to come for a follow-up visit.

The challenge lies in making quality profitable for hospitals instead of being the burden it is now. Hospitals see neither a compulsion nor any significant commercial value in investing in quality, and thus refrain from doing so. The only areas they are forced to invest in are those that the patients can see, like cleanliness, staff courtesy, etc.

Infection rates are again an issue of major concern as they are one of the leading causes of death in a hospital. But many hospitals are not measuring their infection rates, not even in their operation theatres and ICUs. Again, uncomfortable truths could be exposed if this vital data was measured.

This is not to tar all hospitals with the same brush. There are, of course, several hospitals and doctors who, out of a commitment to quality and out of a motivation to improve, measure these indices and act on the data. But for the vast majority of the healthcare system in India, measuring quality is not a priority, certainly not one worth spending on at present.

So, What Next?

It is not enough to just have quality frameworks and policies in place. If we have to progress as a nation, we must measure, monitor and course-correct constantly.

I suggest a seven-point approach:

- Develop a patient-centric culture while creating healthcare policies.
- Ensure that the workforce is well-trained and motivated.
- Focus on public health initiatives that can reduce prevalence of disease and help improve the quality of healthcare delivery.
- Quality is everyone's business, not just the concern of a select few. Every stakeholder must be trained to uphold the highest standards.
- Instil services with empathy and compassion. Focus on the needs of the patient, not on the bottom line.
- Develop systems for timely, accurate and error-free data reporting to ensure stringent measurement. Measure, measure, measure. What cannot be measured cannot be improved.
- Adopt technology for better healthcare delivery.

Quality improvement cannot be brought in by external pressures alone. While stringent laws and legislation help, every stakeholder must uphold the highest of quality standards. The process is continuous and is not a one-off effort. As healthcare professionals, we owe this to our patients and to the community.

5
Does Your Doctor Know Enough?

We had a professor of surgery who, in the politest terms, was not a very good surgeon. But he had a great team of assistants in his unit who would ensure that when the professor entered the operation theatre, a relatively minor surgery (like an Inguinal hernia or hydrocele) would be scheduled on the main table. Some days he would insist on doing a major case. An hour or so into the procedure, as it became messier, he would suddenly remember an important meeting with a minister. This was no surprise to the team as he was politically well connected. Then, the assistants would take over, needing almost an hour just to clean up the mess before starting the actual procedure. Meanwhile, the family of the unfortunate patient would be waiting anxiously.

In bygone years, the physician was akin to God. They were our first and last recourse when we were in pain, and it was believed that they would focus all their energies on providing a cure. Their interest would be entirely on our wellbeing, and we were happy to put them on a pedestal and give them an exalted position in our society.

All that started to change when modern medicine took the commercial route. The physician is still our first resort when in pain but they are no longer a luminous angel. Today's patients are cognizant of the fact that there are very few doctors who may be wholly altruistic, refusing to perceive patients as money-making schemes. Add the ubiquitous 'Dr Google' to the equation and one starts wondering how much the doctor really knows. Do they stay abreast with the latest trends and discoveries? How do you, as a patient, find out the extent of your doctor's knowledge?

What Are Our Expectations from OUR Doctors?

A dipstick survey done by my team revealed that the common expectations a patient has from a doctor are knowledge, quality of care, diagnostic skills, empathy and affordability. The last expectation depends on many factors and may be subjective. Hence, I will address the first four points at greater length.

Knowledge

To quote an article from the Autumn 2015 edition of *Yale Medicine*,[1]

"In the typical adult human—there are 206 bones, at least 700 named muscles, 78 organs, 12 pairs of cranial nerves, and 32 pairs of spinal nerves, and a formidable array of named veins and arteries—all of which, during medical training, a budding doctor will be asked to commit to memory. That, of course, is only the beginning. There are an untold number of procedures to memorize, as well as a host of diseases—currently more than 30,000—to cram into the cerebral cortex, and when the training process is complete, assuming it is ever really done, physicians are expected throughout their careers to dig into their brains' hard drives and retrieve relevant information quickly, effortlessly, and flawlessly ".

Take a moment to mull over this point: no other profession expects so much from an individual. Do you think it is possible for a human being to store and retrieve all this information? Indian education, traditionally, has relied on memorization right from primary schooling, and this carries on to medical education too. But in today's age of artificial intelligence, does a doctor really need to store all the information in their brains? I agree with the article that the focus of learning should be on the methodology and not on memorization.

Quality of care

The quality of care we receive depends to a large extent on how good the physician is. Apart from knowledge, the doctor must have good communication skills, compassion, empathy, an ability to maintain a positive outlook and, of course, honesty and integrity. None of these qualities are part of the medical curriculum. Institutions continue to churn out doctors who may be brimming with knowledge but are severely lacking in other skills.

Diagnostic skills

When a patient meets a doctor, the basic expectation is that they would walk out of the examination room with a diagnosis. As we all know, doctors today rarely arrive at a diagnosis without prescribing a battery of tests. That is not the only factor. Look at your own day, whatever your profession may be. When are you at your most productive? When your mind is fresh and uncluttered or when it is overwhelmed and overloaded? How is it different for doctors? Many of us are aware of the extremely arduous schedules that most doctors in India have. As one of my colleagues said, 'When I started my private practice, I scheduled my working hours as 8–11 a.m. and 5–8 p.m. I naively thought that this would help me juggle my time with my family. My wife is a gynaecologist with uncertain hours, and we wanted someone to be around for our kids. The whole idea crumbled within a few weeks. I tend to stay on till almost 2 p.m. and 11 p.m. on most days. As the only GP in the area, I feel that I owe it to my patients. Sure, I may be generating more income but it has played havoc with my personal life. Most days, I am so sluggish that I am almost on autopilot. And to think that I keep telling my patients to maintain a work–life balance for optimal health. Do as I say, not as I do!'

It is common sense that our productivity in any field of activity depends upon a multitude of factors: how uncluttered our mind is, whether we are in a hurry or not, how physically tired we feel, how alert our brain is, etc. Studies have shown that doctors deliver better results when they see patients in the first half of the day, when the doctor's mind is fresh, than at the end of a long, tiring day when their mind is already cluttered. And God save you if you happen to be the last patient of the day and the doctor's spouse is repeatedly calling to inform them to leave immediately as they are late for a social engagement!

According to me, the accuracy of the diagnosis is effectively dependant on:

- How much of medicine your doctor knows
- The time of the consultation
- The time given for a consultation
- The aptitude and mental makeup of the doctor
- The doctor's ability to communicate their opinion accurately

Empathy

How many of us have seen Indian movies where one of the characters says, 'Doctor, you are like God to us. Please save our parent/child/sibling and we will be indebted to you for life!' Cut to today's era of TV shows like *House MD* and *Grey's Anatomy* where, apart from shenanigans in their personal lives, medicos diagnose and treat serious issues with consummate ease. Most of these shows start with a patient coming in with an inexplicable condition, who is then saved by the brilliance of the medical team. Shows like these tend to deify and venerate medical professionals and justify their exalted status within society.

With so many influences, it is but natural that many doctors develop a God complex. Arrogance becomes second nature to many competent doctors. According to Dr K. Singh,* a well-known and much-respected cardiologist, 'I sometimes think there are two types of people—doctors and non-doctors. As doctors, we are encouraged to arrive at a conclusive diagnosis rather than seek out opinions from other doctors. We are expected to stow away our personal issues and challenges, and attend to the patient. I remember a colleague who operated on a patient within fifteen minutes of facing a severe personal loss. Rescheduling the procedure would have been fatal to the patient and there were no alternative surgeons available immediately. The surgery was successful, and the patient leads a healthy and fulfilling life. Can you blame my colleague for developing a God complex?'

What doctors often forget is that nature heals, and we are just there to assist this process. Often, this can be achieved by leaving the patient alone! As doctors, we have many factors assisting us—our support staff, pharmacological advances, technology—the list is long. To think that it is we and we alone who have cured the patient is sheer foolishness.

Quality of Medical Education

The quality of medical education plays a large role in how much the doctor really knows. Even with almost impossible-to-achieve standards of admission for medical colleges in India, the quality of doctors being churned out is questionable. I maintain that today, it is possible to qualify as a doctor without knowing much about medicine. I have met many young medical graduates who have reinforced this belief. So, where have we gone wrong? Even a few decades ago, only 30–35 per cent of medical students would pass the final MBBS exam. The examination standards were stringent and exacting. Today, most colleges routinely boast of almost 80 per cent pass rate. Does this mean that the current generation is incredibly intelligent and diligent in their academics? I wish it was so! The main reason is that examination standards have fallen drastically. The clinical exams have become progressively—or rather, regressively—less challenging. One must also not ignore the influence of corrupt practices that help churn out less than competent doctors.

Doctors are not tested on how they would manage specific conditions. Problem-oriented medical management is barely touched upon, and examinations tend to focus on theory—most of which will hardly ever be used in clinical practice. It is a tragedy that colleges routinely churn out doctors with little or no knowledge of the protocols on how to manage a patient with chest pain or how to deal with a seizure, or even how to read an ECG or an X-ray. Something as basic as fluid and electrolyte management is a topic that would flummox a sizeable number of specialists and super-specialists!

I graduated with excellent marks and a few prizes and medals to boot. I started my internship with a lot of confidence in my medical abilities. But within a few days, I realized that I was woefully ignorant as to how to manage a patient. The reason? The nuances of managing a patient were not really taught to us at all! While I could reel off twenty-five causes of a symptom or twelve diseases that could cause an abnormal lab value, I simply did not know how to manage the patient, who had any of those conditions. Patient nutrition and fluid balance, a vital part of management, was hardly focused on. It was then that I went back to the basics and relearned most of my medical knowledge, this time from the perspective of applied medicine. I owe a huge debt of gratitude to a teacher of mine, Dr Lakshminarayanan, 'Dr L.N' as he was popularly called, transformed my entire understanding of patient management and taught me to focus on problem-oriented—identifying the problem, or POMD as it is called —medical diagnosis and management in just three months! But how many doctors today have a Dr Lakshminarayanan in their lives to guide them?

Yes, a lot of changes have been made in the curriculum. For instance, the much-needed module on soft skills, Attitude, Ethics and Communication Module (AETCOM), has been implemented in recent years. But is the pace of change rapid enough?

Fatalistic Attitude or Karma?

It is widely acknowledged that the general quality of emerging doctors in India is not what it used to be. There are many new medical colleges, especially in the private sector, where the academic standards are not up to the mark as they just do not have enough clinical material or patients to teach the students. There are far too many students who possibly should not be in a medical school (for reasons of disinterest, parental pressure, poor academic capability, etc.) in the first place getting their degrees. The quality of the faculty is patchy at best. All this means that the doctor who emerges from such a medical school is often a health risk to the patient. Doctors in India have no legal compulsion to keep retraining themselves. They are not audited on any quality-of-care measures; it is pretty much a case of being free to do whatever one wants after the basic qualification is obtained.

All this means that, across India, lakhs of patients could be getting the wrong treatment and incorrect diagnoses, leading to disability or death. Since we are not even measuring the accuracy of the diagnosis and appropriateness of treatment, we simply do not know how big the problem is. There has been strong reluctance to address the issue and take corrective measures. It appears that no one really wants to rake up this matter for fear of opening a can of worms.

The first step would be for the government to commission more studies on a larger scale to continually assess quality measures. This will at least give us scientific evidence of the size and scale of the problem.

The second is to institute and fully integrate protocol-based diagnoses and treatment systems into the teaching programme for medical students.

The third step would be to make doctors take a test every five years to assess if they have updated their skills. Doctors who fail could be given a grace period of a year or two (and multiple attempts) to pass the test. If they still don't, their license could be suspended.

The fourth step could be to use technology with applications like Clinical Decision Support Systems to improve quality-of-care delivery.

All these are vitally important measures for patient's safety.

The tragedy is that our society seems indifferent to the fact that visiting a doctor in most parts of India may actually be dangerous to health. Perhaps it is our belief in destiny or karma that makes us reluctant to fight for this cause. There are very few strong patient bodies or consumer groups that take up these issues with the state or medical associations. A society that does not fight even for something as basic as quality healthcare perhaps deserves the healthcare it gets. The next time you visit your doctor, remember that your odds of getting the right diagnosis and treatment may be an outside shot.

My friend once said, 'I don't understand why you keep talking about reading this and reading that and learning this and learning that. It is not as if there are some ten new bones in the body or that there is a new hidden body part.' I controlled my initial impulse to respond as I was reminded of Mark Twain's immortal quote just in time: 'Never argue with a fool, onlookers may not be able to tell the difference.'

While the human body may not have sprouted wings or extra appendages overnight, there is still much that goes on within it that is still a mystery to us. Apart from that, there are so many newer diseases that have emerged across the world. The COVID-19 pandemic is one such example—doctors are still struggling to learn more about it. Continuous education for a doctor, therefore, is not an option. It is a must, like brushing one's teeth.

Until recently, recertification was not mandatory for doctors in India. In 2002, with approval from the Government of India, the Medical Council of India (MCI) issued a gazette notification, Code of Medical Ethics regulations (Amended up to 8 October 2016), related to professional conduct, etiquette and ethics for registered medical practitioners.[2] Regulation 1.2.3 states:

> A physician should participate in professional meetings as part of a CME programme, for at least 30 hours every five years, organised by reputed professional academic bodies or any other authorised organisations. The compliance of this requirement shall be informed regularly to MCI or SMCs (State Medical Council) as the case may be.

However, this is not yet legally binding and not all doctors apply for recertification. While exact figures are not available, it is suggested that only about 20 per cent of doctors in India follow these requirements.[3]

There are many reasons for this. Even before the COVID-19 pandemic, many doctors in India were severely overworked. It starts from the initial years of their careers, when thirteen- to eighteen-hour workdays are fairly common. It doesn't get easier with passing years. Doctors have to work almost inhuman hours as they progress. Even the most conscientious and punctual doctors would find it difficult to find the hours for CME. Doctors in rural areas are even more challenged to find suitable resources. While online conferences and seminars have made access easier, it is still difficult to find the time. As Dr Joshi,* a doctor working in a rural government hospital, commented, 'Learning requires access, time and, most importantly, a relaxed frame of mind. I don't remember the last time I had time for myself. People tend to forget that we are also humans with family ties. Apart from work, we need to spend time with our loved ones. After all this, finding even an hour in a month for myself is an unaffordable luxury!'

How Do You Decide which Doctor to Go to?

On any given day, I am asked for a referral for a specialist doctor—it may be for a family member, friend, colleague or just a passing acquaintance. People want to know if the doctor is competent and, more importantly, ethical. This led me to wonder how a person chooses a doctor. Asking around for references is a subjective exercise. Today, there are many websites and apps that provide you with ratings of doctors and, supposedly, feedback from genuine patients. But all of us know that these ratings can easily be, and possibly are, manipulated.

Many patients get taken in by the confidence portrayed by their doctor until they realize that a doctor can confidently misdiagnose their condition!

I remember this senior paediatrician, a doctor to children of movie stars and VIPs, who was much sought after. He had an excellent memory and an even better bedside manner. He would remember patients and their history very well. I was taken to him as a child and then happened to see him again after a gap of six years. He impressed my mother by recalling my earlier diagnosis and the medicines he had prescribed then. He even remembered our landline number! We walked out of his cabin, convinced that he was the best doctor under the sun. Years later, after I completed my medical education, I worked as a registrar in the same hospital where he was a consultant. It was then that I realized that behind his amazing bedside manner was an absolute commercial mindset. He would convince parents that their child was gravely ill and he was their saviour. He would admit healthy children to the ICU and the bemused staff would often see his patients running around the ward instead of lying on the ICU beds. If the child had any serious health issue, he would refer them to other specialists and just be the managing doctor. Parents would worship him as, in their eyes, he saved their child from sure death. While we, the staff, knew that he was admitting healthy children, we couldn't do much then. Our careers were at stake, and he was a well-respected senior doctor. But we realized that patients and their family gave more importance to great communication skills and bedside manner rather than knowledge of medicine, which they were in no position to assess.

We assume that when we go to a five-star super specialty hospital we are guaranteed high quality care. Nothing could be further from the truth.

A friend was once admitted to a hospital for an orthopaedic issue. I happened to drop in one morning to the hospital and went over to her room. She was covered with a thick blanket and said that she was feeling very cold. This set alarm bells ringing in my head as I recalled that a couple of years earlier, she had undergone a renal transplant and had multiple complications. I was told that she was seen by a cardiologist, a nephrologist and a physician just a few hours before I met her. All the notes from these doctors were routine but no one had checked why she needed such a thick blanket. I requested the attending nurse to take her temperature and discovered that she was hypothermic—her body temperature was significantly below normal. I then called for the infectious disease doctor, who found out that she had sepsis. Thankfully, we caught it in time and she made a full recovery.

This happened despite the fact that three highly qualified doctors had visited and examined her that very morning! Each specialist checked on their area of speciality and declared she was fine. I call these doctors 'organ doctors', that is, doctors who treat only their respective systems. The cardiologist treats the heart, the nephrologist treats the kidneys, the pulmonologist treats the lungs, etc. In the end, no one treats the patient as a whole. There is hardly any interaction between specialists, and they rarely ever see the patient together.

Once a specialist moves up the ladder in a particular field, they tend to forget the basics of other body systems. This makes the referral system even more pronounced, adding to the number of specialists who are treating a patient. It is not uncommon to see two specialists prescribing drugs that may interact with one another. I have even seen the same drug under two different brand names prescribed by two specialists for the same patient at the same time! Very often, a drug given by one specialist is stopped by another for some valid reason but the original consulting physician who prescribed the drug remains blissfully unaware that the prescription has been modified.

This is compounded by the fact that there is no centralization of medical records. Unlike many Western countries, where any physician can access the patient's medical history with the click of a button, in India, the onus of maintaining medical records largely lies with the patients. Because of this, critical information often falls through the cracks. Doctors simply do not have the time to ask all the relevant questions to arrive at a diagnosis.

Many years ago, I worked at a government PHC in a rural area. There were only two doctors posted there. Every morning, my colleague and I would see around seventy-five patients each in the space of around three hours. That gave us an average of around two and a half minutes per patient. There was hardly any time to get even a basic, let alone detailed, medical history or perform a full physical examination. Added to this, we had to consult with all the outpatient department (OPD) patients in a four-hour timeframe. The second half of the day would be spent on special clinics, immunization programmes or other administrative meetings—all of which are crucial to the training of a doctor.

What would we do? We followed in the footsteps of our seniors. We would ask for the main symptoms, place the stethoscope on the patient's chest (a signal for the patient that they have been examined) and hand over pre-written prescription slips to them. This process was called 'case disposal'. At the end of the day, we would prepare these prescription slips for upper and lower respiratory infections, acute gastroenteritis, otitis media with earache, myalgia and many other common conditions to dispense to patients the next day. Only those who displayed severe symptoms would get more than two minutes of our time and a more detailed examination. I shudder to think about all the diagnoses that we would have missed.

However, the patients had to be seen. It was also important that patients were not kept waiting beyond an hour or so. That was a surefire way of getting into trouble as it would lead to complaints against the doctors and staff of the healthcare centre. No one really knows how many patients suffered because of the two-minute evaluation. Indeed, no one ever kept track of this.

This is the system that continues in thousands of government hospitals across several countries to this day.

So how do doctors get away with it? The answer is that the majority of patients seen in an outpatient clinic would get better with little or no treatment. A very large number of conditions that cause patients to go to a doctor are self-limiting illnesses and get better no matter what treatment is given. This includes the vast majority of respiratory infections, viral fevers, gastroenteritis, other viral illnesses, muscle injuries, etc. A professor of mine would say in jest, 'If you prescribed an analgesic and an antibiotic for four to five days, most of your patients will be cured.'

The Informed Patient

In my early days of practice, I would have the occasional patient who would second guess my diagnosis and would chip in with their own inputs. In the last decade, however, I have the occasional patient who does not do so! Many patients, especially the educated ones, come in with their symptoms and their diagnosis. While this is irritating, there have been times when their inputs have helped, especially with differential diagnoses.

A doctor spends years in training and continues to pore over research to stay up-to-date. So, it feels infuriating if a patient comes up with something after a five-minute internet search. Having said that, we owe it to our patients not to dismiss all their fears but to listen to them. After all, more than in any other field, medicine must rely on shared understanding of complex processes to be optimally effective.[4]

This is true especially in the case of patients with chronic diseases that affect the quality of life but are not life-threatening. I know of many patients who have invested in learning about their condition and are more knowledgeable about their condition than their attending physician. And I know of many arrogant doctors who pooh-pooh their inputs.

I am not suggesting that doctors start taking inputs from the patient but that they be cognizant of the fact that there may be something that the patient knows that the doctor may not have thought of. After all, humility is a virtue when it comes to learning!

A study by the World Bank in 2012[5] in the states of Madhya Pradesh and Delhi found that quacks actually outperformed MBBS doctors. Appalling as it is, this is a sad reflection of the extent of the crisis that we face. While there are pockets of excellence comparable to the best in the world, especially in the metro cities, the vast majority of the country is left at the mercy of poorly trained (or even untrained) and often money-minded doctors.

One of the authors of this study, Jishnu Das, a professor at Georgetown University, describes this puzzle succinctly:[6]

- Most primary care in rural India is provided by informal providers: 77 per cent in rural Madhya Pradesh, 50–80 per cent in other states.
- Even when there is a public-sector clinic in the village, the majority of primary care visits are to informal providers.
- These two facts lay out the fundamental conundrum: (option 1) people are making the best of what they have (one person's 'quack' is another's only hope). Or (option 2) they are being systematically fooled by hundreds of thousands of informal providers running wild in the Indian countryside.

'In fact, the evidence suggests untrained private sector providers (quacks) were better in adhering to the checklist, and no worse in their treatment protocols, than their public sector counterparts (government doctors),' says Das in the study. 'Half of these quacks did not complete secondary education. Many launched their own healthcare practice after being a compounder (assistant to a doctor) for several years.'

While it seems far-fetched that informal health workers provide better healthcare solutions, it is not impossible. I experienced this on my very first night as the on-call duty intern.

A diabetic patient on insulin became drowsy. Not knowing what to do, I called the duty attending physician. Over the phone, he told me to give more insulin. I did. The patient became unconscious. I panicked and called him again. Once more over the phone, he told me he knew the patient's history well and had seen him a few hours ago. It was a case of diabetic keto acidosis and he advised that I should start an insulin drip. Some instinct deep within me was not sure if he was right as the patient's condition had deteriorated after the first shot of insulin. As I was wondering whether to go ahead, in walked a senior (by many years but someone who had not yet completed MBBS). He was what we used to call a chronic additional—someone with several arrears. He took one look at the patient, went through the case records and told me that the patient was in a hypoglycaemic state and urgently needed to be given glucose. My gut told me he could be right. I started a 5 per cent Dextrose drip. Within ten minutes, the patient was conscious and talking normally again.

I still remember that incident like it happened yesterday. What if I had followed the advice of the consultant and started an insulin drip? I could have killed the patient. And on my very first day of call duty too!

This episode highlights the sheer indifference compounded by lack of knowledge of many doctors in the system. While we lament the fact that quacks are destroying the healthcare system, it seems that they are not the only crooks here.

Ask the Right Questions

This is not to say that there aren't any good, knowledgeable and competent doctors. There are thousands and thousands of them! But the aim is to drive home the point that for every such doctor, there may be ten who are not up to the mark and can cause serious harm to your health.

I believe that the system of healthcare practice itself, in some ways, lends itself to medical errors and compromises the quality of care.

You could go to a very knowledgeable physician but still end up with suboptimal care. Most patients do not even know if the doctors know their subject. All they have to go by is the confident manner in which the doctor approaches the patient. The assumption is that the doctor's degree is proof of them knowing medicine. But in the real world, this is not often the case.

Whether your health is so unimportant that it can be left to chance is something that each one of us need to ask ourselves. Why are we not demanding that the quality of care we receive be measured? Why are we not insisting on recertification of doctors as is done in so many countries around the world? Why are we not asking for information on the doctors' track record, success rate, etc.? Some countries provide data on quality indices along with a system that provides an objective method of getting patient feedback. But India has nothing of this sort.

It is time we realize we may be getting suboptimal care and that the reason could be our doctor. Start asking the question 'Does my doctor know enough?' It could lead to you getting better care in the long run.

6

Patient-Centric Care

This is the experience of Lalit Shivtarkar,* a thirty-seven-year-old banker from Chennai: 'My eighty-five-year-old grandmother, like many from her generation, does not have significant health issues, while I pop medicines for cholesterol and hypertension and always watch what I eat! Her rare visits to the doctor were limited to the village doctor, who was not even an MD. The trouble started when she needed a cataract surgery. We convinced her to come to the city for the procedure and stay with us for a few weeks post-surgery. She was not happy about it but realized that she did not have a choice. The procedure went off without a hitch and we were all happy—everyone except my grandmother, that is. She developed acute constipation within a few days of surgery, and nothing seemed to help her. No home remedies, no laxatives, no medicines. Within a month, she was a shadow of her old self and persistently demanded that she be taken back to her home and allowed to die peacefully. Finally, we caved in and took her back home. She summoned the village doctor and spent some time talking to him. He gave her some pills and, within a few days, she was back to her cheerful self. I was thoroughly baffled. The best doctors couldn't help her but this old man managed just that. I sought him out and asked him the same question. He said, "Son, you have to remember that in any treatment, it is important to focus on the patient. Your grandmother has lived all her life in the village and speaks only Marathi. You took her to Chennai, where the eye surgeon could not speak her language. Moreover, she said that he was more focused on making you feel at ease and not her. Since neither he nor the attending staff spoke her language, they compensated by talking to her loudly as though talking to a child. She couldn't understand what was happening to her. And this was repeated with all the doctors who saw her after that. All she needed was reassurance that she was not going blind and becoming dependent on someone else. Since I speak her language, she was comfortable sharing all this with me. I just gave her a mild laxative. Once her fears were allayed, she was okay." He continued, "I see this happen often. Patients need to be understood and comforted. In your grandmother's case, you took her to the best of doctors, but there was no proper channel of communication. After all, illnesses can't be cured only by popping of pills or surgery. Empathy plays a huge role in patient care. Doctors and hospitals must offer patient-centric care! That's where a village doctor like me has an advantage. We really know our patients. But, of course, we will never be recognized the way city doctors are!' He ended with a wry chuckle.

Patient-centric care has become the focus of discussions in healthcare forums. It is one of the key parameters for quality healthcare. The new-age healthcare economy cannot afford to look at patients as cases but instead considers them as consumers. A patient-centric approach benefits not only the patients and the community but will also help the healthcare industry at large.

But isn't the very term an oxymoron? Shouldn't 'patient-centric care' be the very backbone of all healthcare-related activities?

What Makes for a Patient in the First Place?

Words like disease, illness, sickness, etc., are used interchangeably, but there are a few distinctions among them. Professor and General Practitioner Marshall Marinker[1] differentiated these words as follows:

> [Disease] is a pathological process, most often physical as in throat infection, or cancer of the bronchus, sometimes undetermined in origin, as in schizophrenia. The quality which identifies disease is some deviation from a biological norm. There is an objectivity about disease which doctors are able to see, touch, measure, smell. Diseases are valued as the central facts in the medical view […]

> Illness is a feeling, an experience of unhealth which is entirely personal, interior to the person of the patient. Often it accompanies disease, but the disease may be undeclared, as in the early stages of cancer or tuberculosis or diabetes. Sometimes illness exists where no disease can be found. Traditional medical education has made the deafening silence of illness-in-the-absence-of-disease unbearable to the clinician. The patient can offer the doctor nothing to satisfy their senses—he can only bring messages of pain to the doctor, from an underworld of experience shut off forever from the clinical gaze […]
>
> Sickness is the external and public mode of unhealth. Sickness is a social role, a status, a negotiated position in the world, a bargain struck between the person henceforward called 'sick', and a society which is prepared to recognize and sustain him. The security of this role depends on a number of factors, not least the possession of that much 'treasured' gift, the disease […]
>
> To become a patient is to establish a healing relationship with another who articulates society's willingness and capability to help.

In this case, the medical community represents society. How many of us continue to meet doctors even after we no longer have any demonstrable disease or complaints of illness or sickness?

Ill health is a highly personal experience that depends on how the person views their condition and the consequences of the ailment. Ill health brings a lot of changes including, but not limited to, alienation from their own body, disrupted ordinary life, removal from social roles and obligations, and disturbed relationships with family, work colleagues and friends.[2] Irrespective of whether it is an acute or chronic condition, the person needs to understand their new reality and make a series of changes in their life. These changes do not just affect the individual but also their social group and environment.

But the concept of good health is a complex issue in itself. It is not simply the absence of disease, sickness or illness. I remember allaying my grandmother's fears when she used to complain about vague aches and pains as part of the ageing process. It was not till she retorted one day, 'Then maybe that is my sickness! Why don't you take my complaints seriously?', that this point was driven home. A person can feel unwell even in the absence of disease and conversely can be completely asymptomatic even when diseased. Health is not merely a physical state but—as we are increasingly realizing—also a mental and emotional one.

The health of an individual is not just internal, or only dependent on how they feel. Their environment—physical, social as well as emotional environment—plays a huge role in this aspect, as does their ability to adapt and integrate into their life context.[3] The 'normality' of health also needs to be looked at in the context of gender, geographical location, living conditions, age, etc. Health is subjective and will differ even between members of the same family—it can be different even among identical twins! It is clear that the concept of ill health is not as simple as it sounds. And a physician or healthcare attendant plays an important role in how the person perceives their health.

The Doctor–Patient Relationship

The doctor–patient relationship is remarkable for its centrality during life-altering and meaningful times in a person's life, such as birth and death, as well as periods of severe illness and healing.[4] Since time immemorial, this relationship has been the very foundation of healthcare.

> This relationship is based on four elements:[5,6,7]
>
> - Mutual knowledge: how well the doctor knows the patient and how well the patient knows the doctor
> - Trust: the patient's trust in the doctor's competence and care, and the doctor's trust that the patient is honest in reporting their symptoms
> - Loyalty: the patient's willingness to forgive a doctor for minor inconveniences (commuting distance, time spent in the waiting room, etc.) and the doctor's commitment to never abandon a patient
> - Regard: the patient feeling that the doctor is on 'their side' and treats them as a unique individual

These aspects influence how the patient feels during and after the consultation. It is interesting to note that a cure is not an aspect that influences this experience. Nagpur-based architect Piya Sharma* echoes this sentiment: 'I was diagnosed with rheumatoid arthritis when I was in my early thirties. I remember the first doctor who diagnosed me—he was very curt and basically informed me that I will be a lifelong patient and will have a poor quality of life. Imagine my plight—I was a young mother, doing well in my career and this diagnosis came as a bolt of lightning. I just sunk deep into depression and wanted to curl up and die. I was then referred to another rheumatologist who basically said the same thing—but in a completely different way. He encouraged me to join a support group and focus on what I can do rather than what cannot be done. He gave me a lot of literature to read up on and connected me with a physiotherapist who helped me with a proper exercise routine. He connected me to a wellness coach who enabled me with the tools to manage my anxiety and worries. He encouraged me to take a sabbatical from work and focus on my health. I returned to work after a year and did very well in my career. Yes, I am on medication, and I do have good and bad days, but I really believe that if I had continued with my first doctor, I would have been either wheelchair-bound, or worse, killed myself.'

Hungarian psychoanalyst Michael Balint claimed that 'the most powerful therapeutic tool the doctor possessed was himself or herself'.[8] Way back in 1964, he encouraged doctors to look past physical signs and symptoms and focus on the patient's unique psychological and social context, thereby allowing them to understand the 'real' reason for the consultation. In a way, this can be considered as the basis of patient-centred care.

Simply put, the patient-centred care approach believes that the process of healing depends not only on accurate diagnosis and various medical treatments, but also on knowing the patient as a person. This approach is not new. If we look at the evolution of medicine, knowing the patient was considered the first step to curing them. With the advent of diagnostic tests and the commercialization of healthcare, the focus has shifted to making money. Multiple research projects and surveys conclude that patients want doctors who appear interested, listen well, explain clearly, are open to discussion and involve the patient in decision-making.

The Institute of Medicine defines patient-centred care as 'providing care that is respectful of, and responsive to, individual patient preferences, needs and values, and ensuring that patient values guide all clinical decisions'.[7]

In patient-centred care, all healthcare decisions are made based on the patient's specific needs and their desired health outcomes. Patients do not just follow medical instructions blindly but are true partners in their treatment. Further, treatment is based not only on the clinical perspective, but also on emotional, mental, spiritual, social and financial perspectives. The goal of patient-centred care is best explained by Balint:[8] 'to understand the complaints offered by the patient, and the symptoms and signs found by the doctor, not only in terms of illnesses, but also as expressions of the patient's unique individuality, their conflicts and problems'.

Effective communication, then, is the cornerstone of this approach. But how can this be achieved if the doctor has little time or is preoccupied during the consultation? It is also important to note that the success of this approach is dependent on other factors like accessibility, affordability and quality of healthcare.

Medical treatment is not limited only to the doctor–patient interaction. It begins much before a person actually seeks out a doctor. Public health initiatives to prevent illnesses, access to medical care, ease of appointment, waiting time in the clinic are all part of this process. Advertising professional Rhea Sampat* says, ' I had moved into a new city as a first-time mother. My son developed fever and loose motions. Even a sip of water would lead to a watery bowel movement. My husband was travelling, and I sought help from the neighbours who advised various home remedies. But my son's condition didn't improve. By the evening, I was exhausted and terrified. I called the office of a paediatrician, who was highly recommended by the neighbours. The receptionist curtly told me that the slots for that evening were filled up and the doctor does not see walk-in patients, especially the new ones. I requested for the first slot the next morning. Her reply? "Well, as a policy, we do not give appointments the previous day. You need to call in the morning and fix an appointment."

I replied that it was very difficult to get through as the phone lines are constantly busy and it would be difficult for me to keep dialling while tending to my son (this was before the mobile phone era!). I pleaded with her to give me the first slot (at 9 a.m.) and assured her that I would be there fifteen minutes before the appointment. All my entreaties fell on deaf ears, and she kept echoing that policies cannot be changed for everyone. I was angry and humiliated, but I did not have any option, but to just take my unwell son the next morning and plonk myself at the clinic by 8.45 a.m. But even then, I had to wait for two hours before the doctor could see us. The doctor arrived only by 10 a.m. and then he took in a few other patients who had come in before me. My son had three more episodes of loose stools by then and every time, I had to manage changing a wriggling baby in a smelly, not very hygienic toilet. When I finally met the doctor, he spent two minutes with us and handed a pre-printed form to me and refused to answer any questions and literally shooed me out of his office. He had the temerity to say that he had patients with more serious cases waiting. I agree that for him, it may not be a crisis, but I was a nervous wreck. Shouldn't a doctor have some empathy for the patient and the immediate caregiver? If he doesn't have the time, he could have had a nurse answer my queries and clear my doubts. My son did recover soon, and I also learned more as a mother and did not panic as much the next time. But a compassionate approach would have gone a long way that day.

If this was the treatment meted out to someone like me, an educated well-to-do woman, I shudder to think how the poor are treated in this country.'

I am frequently told that to expect patient-centred care in a country where millions still lack access to any form of healthcare at all is like asking for the moon. My counterpoint is that this is the same country that has a Mars mission. If that can be done, why can't I ask for the moon and get it too?

How can you only talk about wanting to be best in the world without taking concrete actions? The patient-centred care approach is the first step towards improving the quality of healthcare delivery. We need to have deep respect for patients as unique individuals and provide care that is suited to them. Patients must be listened to and respected, and their wishes honoured. After all, it is their health and their lives at stake. Of course, this does not imply that the patient's every whim must be pandered to. It means that the attending doctor understands the patient's unique circumstances and plans the treatment accordingly.

Consider the experience of Sameer Kamat,* a businessman from Indore: 'My doctor does not share some of my medical reports with me. He insists on my going to a particular testing centre for all my tests and the diagnostic test results are sent to him directly. He then decides on the treatment plan without discussing any options with me.

Once, when I had continuous back pain, he recommended surgery after X-rays and MRIs and—no surprises—referred the surgeon too! I wanted a second opinion before any invasive procedure but my doctor simply refused to share the images. His secretary claimed that as a policy, the clinic maintains all the patient records. Finally, I had to repeat all the tests at another centre. It was expensive but it was better than surgery. The next doctor I went to recommended physiotherapy and postural corrections, and within a few months, I was much better. I exercise religiously and ensure that I maintain proper posture, etc. But even if I had needed surgery, don't I have the right to my own medical records? It is my body, my life, and I am paying for it!'

I know of many doctors who follow this practice of withholding the records of their patients. One reason behind this is that some doctors feel that the patients do not maintain their records properly and many forget to bring them when they arrive for consultations. While this may be true, another unsaid reason is to avoid losing patients to other doctors.

Research has shown that health outcomes are much more promising when the patient feels respected, involved and engaged in their treatment.[9] Unlike the earlier days when a patient had little recourse but to follow what the doctor prescribed, most patients today want to know exactly why a certain course of action is prescribed. The ability to communicate empathetically with patients is a must in doctors.

Genuine face-to-face patient interaction is often missed out by many busy doctors and medical care teams. However, to a patient who is already scared, this is the crucial factor that affects their healing process. Ameetha Nambiar,* a fifty-six-year-old homemaker, says, 'I was admitted to the hospital for a tumour removal in the liver. It had come up during some routine tests, and further tests revealed the tumour, so there was no other option but to remove it. Throughout the process, the doctor spoke to my husband and not to me. Even when I asked questions, he would either ignore them or maintain eye contact with my husband. I was so frustrated. At night, this frustration would turn to fear. Maybe the doctor knows that I am dying? Maybe that's why he can't look at me directly? The constant stress increased my blood pressure and the stress eating led to unnecessary weight gain. Thank God that the tumour was benign, and I was okay. But I would never recommend that doctor to anyone. Was I just a case to him?' Arguably, her recovery would have been much faster if her stress levels had been down.

In an effort to enhance the patient experience, many hospitals have refurbished their appearance to resemble that of a hotel. However, this does not necessarily promise a patient-centred approach. Larger hospitals—especially corporate hospitals—tend to focus on efficiencies and have invested heavily in technology for the same. To quote Dr Roopa Mahesh,* 'Having trained in the US, I have always advocated adopting a patient-centred approach in my clinic. It was not till I was myself a patient did I really understand its true value. I was diagnosed with early-stage oesophageal cancer, and surgery was the first line of treatment. As a gynaecologist, I had a better knowledge of cancer than a layperson. But as the saying goes, doctors are the worst patients. I had handled many complicated births successfully, but when it came to my own surgery, I was extremely apprehensive. My surgeon was the best in the country. Highly skilled but with an extremely curt bedside manner. While I am extremely thankful for his expertise that ensured that the tumour was removed completely with no other complications, I am more grateful to the nurses who held my hand during my darkest hours. I also am grateful to the junior doctors who on their daily rounds would find time to talk to me—not as a colleague, but as a patient who is scared and worried.'

One Step Further: People/Person-Centred Care

While the terms 'patient-centred' and 'person-centred' are used interchangeably, there is a subtle difference. When the term 'patient' is used, there is an unconscious shift of power to the medical professional, and this does not augur well for an equal relationship.

> The fundamental difference between the two terms is the purpose behind them:[10]
>
> ⊕ The main goal of patient-centredness is the functional life of the patient.
> ⊕ The main goal of person-centredness is the meaningful life of the patient.

Even the WHO has accepted the need for patient-centeredness as an important global issue and identified it as one of the six attributes of quality healthcare, the others being safety, timeliness, effectiveness, efficiency and equity.[11]

But some of the broader health challenges are better met by a people-centred approach, where it is acknowledged that it is essential to empower people to manage and protect their own health. It is also imperative to consider the needs of people working in the healthcare setting.

A people-centred approach then ensures an equal balance of power among all the stakeholders—the person, community and the healthcare providers.

The first step in achieving this is to retrain our medical professionals. Doctors and other healthcare providers must be trained in communicating and listening. They need to speak in a language that the patient can understand, and their body language should match their verbal communication. It is also essential for them to check the patient's understanding of the treatment protocol.

Efforts have to be made to spend sufficient time while consulting with the patient. The medical professional has to understand that the person walking into their consultation room plays multiple roles that may affect the way they seek medical care. For example, a busy mother who has to juggle a family and career may find it difficult to take time for self-care, which may adversely affect her recovery. There would be times when the doctor is at a complete loss as to what is wrong with the patient. At these times, it is important to be open to learning and reaching out to other colleagues who can help.

Many a time, doctors deliver unpleasant news in a very unorganized way, which leaves patients bewildered and uncertain. This affects the patient's trust in the doctor. As mentioned earlier, it is important to treat the patient as an adult and talk *to* them and not *at* them. In cases of chronic ailments, it would be helpful to refer the patient to suitable support services. Often, the patient is left flabbergasted with the diagnosis and the proposed treatment plan. If it is not a medical emergency, it is better to give the patient some time to understand and accept the treatment plan.

Doctors must understand that when patients walk into their room, they are often scared and intimidated. The onus of setting them at ease lies solely on the medical team. While the doctor may be at ease asking probing and personal questions that are relevant for diagnosis, the patient may not always be forthcoming.

Technology can play a large role in ensuring person-centred care. A robust documentation system will help in the quick retrieval of the patient's history, even if there is a change in the attending doctor.

Is This an Unachievable Dream for India?

As a nation, we can no longer hide under the excuse that we are a third-world country and have few resources for patient-centred care. We have taken giant strides in many other fields, and healthcare needs to have the same kind of importance.

With the increase in the percentage of chronic diseases, patient-centred care is a necessity. It is important to create a high level of health literacy amongst people through mass media campaigns and strong health education programmes from a young age. Apart from medical care, there needs to be ancillary training programmes on managing chronic diseases. Creation of support groups and community level organizations can also help people manage their health better.

Medical professionals must be taught about people-centred approaches from the time they enter medical school. Healthcare providers must ensure a safe and comfortable space for patients and practitioners alike. Incentives must be provided for ethical and compassionate services. Adoption of appropriate technology will help in monitoring and evaluating the performance of the staff. I reiterate that investing in public health will go a long way in ensuring people-centred care.

7

Should Healthcare Be a For-Profit Industry?

Mariam was a fifty-year-old single parent of two teenage daughters, struggling to eke out a living on her meagre salary as a primary school teacher. She was the sole breadwinner. Fate struck again when she was diagnosed with breast cancer. The silver lining was that though it was at a late stage, the cancer was treatable. She started her treatment at a privately-owned oncology centre. The tumour was removed after an operation, and she was recommended a course of chemotherapy. Having exhausted her scanty funds on the surgery and a few cycles of chemotherapy, she decided to temporarily pause the chemo sessions. When the attending doctor tried to change her decision, she said, 'I have two daughters. I need to educate them and ensure that they are financially independent. How can I borrow money for my treatment when there are mounting college fees? My elder daughter has only one more year to graduate and once she starts earning, I can restart my treatment.'

Unfortunately, without timely chemo, the disease spread and she succumbed to it.

In a country like India, almost 30 per cent of patients discontinue their cancer treatment simply because of lack of funds. Often, families are torn between spending the meagre resources they have on the living or the dying. This is not unique to India. Medical treatment is expensive and the government hospitals that offer free treatment do not inspire trust. These hospitals are poorly staffed, inadequately equipped and, more importantly, there is an absolute lack of empathy in many of the staff in these hospitals.

On the other side of the spectrum, we have swanky corporate hospitals which promise the best of care—provided you have the financial bandwidth.

Where does that leave lakhs of Indians who desperately need medical assistance? Private hospitals operate with an eye on profit and not on care.

Profit is not a bad word, but profiting from human pain and suffering as the healthcare industry does has a particularly unpleasant feel to it. You may argue that the money is being made through reducing human suffering by treating illnesses. But, at the end of the day, if that result is achieved by bankrupting families and driving them below the poverty line, it is simply unacceptable.

As in any other business, hospitals make profits when income exceeds expenditure. And like all businesses, the management team keeps a close watch on both these aspects. So, how does the team ensure higher revenues? Definitely not on one-off doctor consultations! The moolah really flows in from all that is prescribed to the patient after the consult.

Business is generated when the attending doctor orders tests or procedures, admits the patient for a hospital stay or refers them to other specialists at the same hospital or chain of hospitals.

If all patients were seen by doctors and simply sent home with a prescription, most hospitals would go broke!

Whenever someone complains about the high cost of medical care, there is always a counter-suggestion: 'Why don't you go to a government hospital? There, the treatment is either free or highly subsidized!'

Really? In the developed countries of the Western world, there may be little difference between the functioning of a for-profit and a non-profit hospital. But across large parts of the developing world, non-profit hospitals often have poorer infrastructure and pay lower salaries to the medical staff. As a result, they are unable to attract and retain the best talent. The government hospitals are overcrowded, and the less said about their treatment protocols, the better. Why would someone willingly seek treatment at such a facility? Even if it is financially draining, we tend to seek the best medical care available for our loved ones.

For all purposes, the industry is classified under the 'service' sector. But there ends the similarity with other businesses under the same umbrella. In this industry, good quality service or personnel does not necessarily lead to the best results.

Here are a few other differences:

Can You Choose the Doctor?

Suppose you have a medical emergency. There is not much time to think; you will be taken to the closest hospital and be relegated to the care of the doctor-on-call. Other factors like affordability and regulations also play important roles in determining the healthcare provider.

Great Service! Will You Go Back?

Rajendra* was rushed to the hospital after an accident that resulted in a fracture. He was quickly attended to; the doctors performed a surgery and inserted a plate to fix his bone. After a few days, he was discharged. He went for a review after a couple of weeks and another after a month. Thereafter, he was given the all clear. He was extremely satisfied with the quality of care but he is unlikely to be a repeat customer to the orthopaedic department of that hospital unless, God forbid, he has another fracture, of course! This is different from, say, buying a phone. Rajendra may buy a new iPhone every other year if he is satisfied with its quality and services.

Diagnosis or Treatment: What Costs More?

Suppose your refrigerator is malfunctioning. The manufacturer may charge a minimum amount to cover the cost of diagnosis. The bulk of the bill amount is always paid only for the solution. However, in the case of healthcare, a large portion of the bill may be the charges for the diagnostic tests!

Given these factors, it is anybody's guess as to where the incentive lies for healthcare professionals: maximizing revenues from a single visit or investing in building customer goodwill!

How Does a Doctor Generate Revenue?

The first way is through consultations, of course. Meeting patients and addressing their concerns is the primary job of a doctor. However, the revenue generated from a single patient visit is not very high. Often, doctors are trained by their employers to maximize revenues during the acute phase of illness of a patient.

Not many doctors want to take the risk of letting nature take its course and the patient recovering on their own. Imagine the loss of revenue to the doctor and, more importantly, to the hospital!

So, instead of adopting a conservative line of treatment, the doctor may then refer the patient for tests and other diagnostic procedures in the initial phase, when the patient is acutely ill. While many of these tests are of course required to make the diagnosis early, it is at this phase that several unnecessary ones are also ordered—ensuring significant revenues to the hospital.

Surgical procedures are another way of increasing revenues. It is not just the procedure that brings in the revenues but also the many other ancillary services. Many hospitals tend to charge the patient based on the type of room they choose. If you are in a single deluxe room, you pay more for all services and not just for the comfort of the room. Everything, including the food charges, are higher as compared to a bed in a general ward of the same hospital.

Many hospitals have targets for the number of days a patient should be in the hospital as they have a limited number of beds. Hence, doctors are encouraged to have short-stay patients, if beds are in short supply, to maximize revenue yield per bed. Revenue tends to dry up if a patient merely occupies the room and does not need more extensive testing or further procedures. Obviously, it makes commercial sense for a hospital to admit a new patient to that room, ensuring higher revenues (until that patient too hits the base room rent levels and the cycle continues).

On the other hand, if the hospital has low occupancy rates, the doctors may be encouraged to delay discharging the patient—thereby adding to the overall revenues of the hospital.

> ### How Are Doctors Compensated?
>
> The most common compensation structures for doctors are:
>
> - 100 per cent Salary Model: The doctor is paid a fixed salary.
> - Salary Plus Incentive Model: A portion of salary is fixed, and the rest is in the form of incentives based on revenue generated by the doctor or the department.
> - Equal Shares Model: Whatever income is generated by the practice, after deducting all expenses, is paid out equally to all the doctors in the practice.
> - Pure Productivity Model: Doctors earn a share of whatever revenue is generated by them.
>
> As you can see, there is an element of incentive or variable pay for doctors. Generally, the more senior a doctor, the higher the incentives. Isn't it natural that when a hospital incentivizes a doctor, it changes the way the doctor thinks and works? Wouldn't they find it exceedingly difficult to put the patient's interests first?

When Profit Becomes a Four-Letter Word!

$$\text{Profit} = \text{Selling Price} - \text{Cost Price}$$

This is the simple formula to calculate profit. My opinion is that hospitals should make profits—provided they put the interests of the patients first. But many hospitals take this focus on profit to ridiculous heights. Be it price markups on services rendered or differential pricing on medicines, there are enough examples to fill a whole book! Due to paucity of space, I cite only a few examples here.

Price markups

Price markups are one of the most common methods to increase revenue.

One such example is that of intravenous (IV) fluids, sterile saline water that is administered to the patient as part of their treatment. It is a basic component of emergency treatment. It is also one of the least expensive treatments—just not for the patient!

In my early years as a doctor in a semi-private hospital, a bag of IV fluids would be supplied to the in-house pharmacy at ₹8 a bag. This would be sold to the patient at ₹32 a bag, which is a margin of a whopping 400 per cent!

Another example is the billing of personal protective equipment (PPE) kits. These kits are used by medical professionals while treating patients with highly infectious diseases. Patients discharged after being treated for COVID-19 are billed for the cost of these kits. Fair enough.

But each patient in the ward would be charged for the PPE kit even when the nurses or doctors do not change their kit for every patient. If there are ten patients in a ward, each pays ₹2,000 per day for the kit. With a minimum hospitalization of ten days, the hospital makes ₹20,000 per patient, and for a ward of ten patients, they earn a revenue of ₹2 lakh over the duration of the patients' stay—on PPE kits alone! And the cost to the hospital? Most likely, less than ₹25,000—you don't need to be a mathematician to figure out the profit margins!

Same pill, different price

Medication is an important component of your treatment process, and this is another area where hospitals make money. When it comes to medicines, there are different brands of the same drug. They may have the same composition and dosage and are meant for the same condition. They also have the same effects (and side-effects!), but different pharmaceutical companies brand them differently and price them differently too.

This is best illustrated with an example.

Atenolol is a generic drug. It is a beta blocker that is used to treat high blood pressure and irregular heartbeats, or arrhythmia. It has been around for decades and is off patent, which means that pretty much anyone can manufacture it. This is sold by multiple pharmaceutical companies under different brand names. And the price ranges from ₹9.48 (FDC Limited) to ₹33.52 (Cipla) for a strip of 50mg tablets. Now, why would the same off-patent medicine have such a wide variation in price is anybody's guess. For obvious reasons, doctors are persuaded to prescribe the higher priced drugs and the clueless patient has no other choice but to buy the prescribed brand.

A 2018 article throws light on the profit margins made by hospitals in India[1] on a few medical consumables and drugs. Hospitals make up to 1,737 per cent profit on Romson's three-way stopcock (bivalve) and 1,208 per cent profit on Lifelong's disposable syringes. If the hospital uses Samarth Pharma's Adrenor injection (used in heart arrest and allergy), the profit margin is a sweet 1,192 per cent. Treating a bacterial infection? Acumentis healthcare's Todaycef injection gives a profit margin of 966 per cent! And with Neon's Dotamin (used in cardiac decompensation), the hospital makes a profit margin of 914 per cent.

Time to Ponder

When a doctor is examining you in their clinic, what do we expect to be uppermost in their mind? That they are primarily concerned about us, their patients. Whether it is an emergency visit, regular checkups, or treatment for a particular ailment, we expect our doctors and hospitals to offer us the best treatment option possible—preferably without bankrupting us!

Let me now present the perspective of the attending doctor. They are employees at the hospital who are expected to generate revenues for it. As we saw earlier, the doctor has zero incentive to just examine you and say there is nothing seriously wrong, prescribe an over-the-counter medicine and send you home.

It makes better financial sense to order tests and procedures, and you end up paying for both necessary as well as unnecessary tests.

Of course, doctors take the Hippocratic oath and promise to put patients first, and many of them genuinely do. But human nature being what it is, it is naive to expect thousands of healthcare professionals to completely let go of their drive to seek profit or money. The fault is not theirs but in the system that, instead of aligning their interests with that of their patients, pits them against each other.

Isn't it time to realign the interests of all the players in healthcare—hospitals, doctors and patients?

The Problem with For-Profit Hospitals

Are you aware that at least half of the world's population cannot obtain essential health services? And the numbers of households that are pushed into poverty because of medical expenses is mind-boggling!

Is it not a grotesque inequality that the very right to life itself is linked to economic capability? Is this not an unacceptable situation? While we have people protesting for all kinds of equal rights, why have we accepted with a shrug that this is how it will be?

We are not talking of free healthcare for all here, while that also deserves a more serious discussion. Every industry has costs, and the healthcare industry, with its huge investments on medical technologies and personnel, has more than its fair share. These costs need to be recovered and the healthcare staff need to be paid well too. However, what we are exploring here is whether greed, rather than necessity, should be allowed to decide who lives and who dies. To me, that seems perverse. When the doctor has been drilled to look at the profit motive, it is only natural that they imbibe this desire to seek profits over patient care in all their interactions with the patient.

The modern-day for-profit hospital is often run like a ruthless corporation. The balance sheet is carefully scrutinized, and every heading is analysed to maximize revenue generation. While this may be a good business practice, this bothers me at many levels. I have seen hospitals close down medical services as they were not deemed 'profitable'. I have also seen doctors in these hospitals peddle unnecessary services only because they are profitable and make more business sense. Hospitals should provide care without prejudice, but that is not necessarily the outlook of many hospitals today. The paying customer often gets precedence over someone who may be in urgent need of medical care.

In the last twenty years, many countries have witnessed a growth in corporate private hospitals, or hospitals owned by large business groups. With this emerged a new breed of hospital management professionals—great strategists and marketing professionals who dictate how the hospital should be run.

Consider the compensation packages of healthcare CEOs. These are women and men with great business acumen who are compensated handsomely for ensuring high returns to the investors. They ensure that the hospital brings in enough profits to justify their mind-boggling compensation packages.

According to a CEO of a big corporate hospital in Mumbai, who spoke to me on the condition of anonymity, 'I have been hired to increase the profits of the hospital. My job depends on that and not on the number of patients the hospital cures or the number of students we teach. With such a clear mandate, how can I not be ruthless when it comes to upselling to patients?'

These hospitals tend to gobble up small clinics and private practice groups with many incentives. The nexus between politics and business is even more prevalent in the healthcare sector. Greasing the hands of powerful politicians helps in getting special privileges.

In India, large for-profit corporate hospitals get huge import duty exemptions on medical equipment. This is on the condition that the hospitals provide free or concessional services to a certain percentage of patients—a condition that is flouted with impunity. The larger hospitals in a town also tend to form a cartel, giving the patient truly little to choose from when it comes to costs of tests or procedures.

Profits are needed to keep hospitals open. Profits help hospitals serve patients who cannot pay. Profits help hospitals invest in better infrastructure. Profits help hospital employees earn a decent wage. Profits are the very basis of any business.

But when a doctor sees a patient, they must have only one interest in mind: the best interest of the patient. Anything else that comes into the equation is a corruption of their intent in some form.

Why Do I BELIEVE that Hospitals Be Not for Profit?

A caveat: when I talk about nonprofit, I refer to organizations in the developing world which are managed like an actual nonprofit, and not to those giant entities in countries like the US that are nonprofit institutions only on paper.

If you are a walk-in patient seeking basic medical care, you may not find much of a difference between a good quality nonprofit and for-profit hospital. Both follow all required medical protocols, have professional and qualified staff, and offer medical care to the patient. It is what happens behind the scenes that sets these two entities apart.

Most private hospitals, whether non-profit or for-profit, function similarly. The bottom line matters for both these types of institutions. Unlike in a public or charitable hospital, the doctor, here, has a fiscal accountability apart from providing quality care.

Obviously, someone has to pay for healthcare costs—the industry cannot survive without funds. But whether it is the government or insurance companies, it is ultimately us, taxpaying citizens, who are directly or indirectly footing the bill. That's when we need to ask a few questions:

- At the end of the day, to whom is the hospital primarily responsible?
- Is it to the owners and shareholders who pay the salaries or is it to the patients they treat?

- Are patients merely the medium to satisfy the shareholders?

It is indeed difficult for a doctor on a variable compensation structure not to think of money in their dealings with their patients.

I maintain that doctors need to be paid fixed salaries which do not vary based on the number of surgeries or procedures they do. That is largely the case in health systems run by governments in many countries. While this may leave a lesser incentive for a doctor to excel, it should go a long way in managing healthcare costs and preserving the interests of the patient.

Hospitals could also be paid based on outcomes and not diagnoses and treatment procedures. With the famous Indian propensity for jugaad, this may lead to fudging of statistics, which, I believe, would be a more manageable problem. At least there would be some incentive in the system for the hospital and the doctor to promote health and keep people healthy.

Paying hospitals for outcomes rather than procedures is a common-sense way of getting the medical community to focus on doing what is in the patients' interest rather than their own. For instance, if a hospital was to be paid a sum for treating a cardiac patient—and this payment was to be linked to measurable outcomes in terms of morbidity (symptom relief and quality of life indices) and mortality (and not just on the tests performed or surgeries done)—there would be a strong incentive to do the right thing and not simply build a case for expensive procedures and treatment options. With outcome-based compensation almost unheard of in the developing world, or even in many parts of the Western world, it is an option that surely appears to be worth a try.

Another radical option would be to try and bypass the medical industry in the initial process of healthcare delivery, using AI supported expert systems to help in the screening of populations. Only those who are identified to have specific organic illnesses would then be referred for further treatment. With newer expert systems coming to the fore, this could prove to be an option that holds great promise, especially as it is a model that is replicable on a mass scale. Potentially, the best screening tools available in the world could then be made accessible to a poor villager in the remotest corner of the country. Wouldn't this be a better option than the poorly trained and overburdened general practitioner they may otherwise have access to?

> In my opinion, an ideal nonprofit hospital would be one where:
>
> - Doctors and staff are paid a fixed salary and are not incentivized on the basis of procedures, diagnostic tests or any other criteria.
> - Tests and procedures are priced at cost, with a reasonable profit margin.

> - Tariffs are standard across the institution except for room rent.
> - Drugs are sold at discounted prices based on the discounts received from distributors and not at MRP.
> - Support is sought from the community and corporates in the region to help sustain growth.
> - Transparency is maintained across all functions and departments in the hospital.

Whatever the model considered, it is time that the healthcare industry starts to take a hard look at itself and explore alternate models of quality care delivery, and not only focus on profits. Unaffordable for the vast majority of the world, the industry has the option of voluntarily participating in the change before change is thrust on it. After all, how long can the industry operate on the infamous catchphrase 'Kill him if you will, but please, please bill him'?

8

Is Big Pharma Influencing Your Treatment?

Lopa Goswami* is a worried woman. Her entire household seems to be surviving on medication. Her fifty-six-year-old husband is on medications for controlling cholesterol and hypertension, she is on hormone replacement therapy for menopause, her twenty-three-year-old son is on medication for social anxiety disorder and her twenty-year-old daughter has been on medications for Attention-Deficit/Hyperactivity Disorder (ADHD) since she was sixteen. 'Whenever I visit India, I am amazed that my parents who are well into their eighties are not on any medication. They, in turn, wonder at the number of medications we have. I cannot even explain these conditions to them. I am the laughing stock of my brother and sister. They call me the "sick Amrikawali" as they think that all these diseases are only in the US.' She however was in for a shock when, on her 2022 visit to India, discovered that her fifteen-year-old niece was under treatment for depression, her fifty-one-year-old sister-in-law was on medications for osteoporosis, and her sixty-two-year-old brother was on medication for irritable bowel syndrome. 'While these diseases are quite common in the US, I did not realize that these are becoming increasingly common in India too. I am not even sure if these are real conditions or if we are just adding to the revenues of the pharma companies. What is frightening is that once we start on most of these medications, we cannot quit them cold turkey. These medications also have many side-effects which are treated with more medications. It is a vicious circle, one which we can't seem to escape.'

Lopa should be worried. I am not dismissing the existence of these conditions or the real suffering of people with these conditions. But I do question the pill-popping solutions for all conditions. How many of these patients are suffering from real diseases and how many are victims of disease mongering, where the definition of these conditions has been broadened by pharmaceutical companies with profit in mind?

Any discussion on healthcare would be incomplete without a mention of how Big Pharma, a term used to denote the global pharmaceutical industry, affects the way doctors prescribe—or rather push—medications irrespective of the needs of the patient.

Pharma companies spend a lot of money on research and, technically, any drug that is developed needs to go through intensive checks and clinical trials before they are launched. The clinical trials are supposed to be well-monitored and done with the complete consent of the participant. But companies are known to conduct dodgy trials in India, where the laws are not as rigid as in Western countries. Often, the participants are akin to hapless lab rats who have been coerced into the trial.

In this chapter, I address all these issues and answer the question: how do pharmaceutical companies affect your healthcare?

What Is Disease Mongering?

Shobhana Lakshman* is a psychotherapist based in Bengaluru. She largely works with young adults and, over the last twenty odd years, has built quite a bit of expertise in the area of mental health of that age group. When I spoke to her, she said, 'I remember that in my early years as a therapist, seeing a therapist was considered a social stigma. This has changed over the years. It is more acceptable to see a therapist now. As a therapist, I do not prescribe medications. If I think that a particular client needs medical help, I refer them to a psychiatrist. In my experience, only a small percentage of my clients need pharmacological help. The others benefit from other forms of therapy. What is alarming is the number of young professionals who self-diagnose themselves and pester me for references. One of the common diagnoses they come up with is social anxiety disorder. This is a serious condition that cripples the affected individual and isolates them socially. However, for most of those who complain of this, the common symptoms are nothing but shyness and low self-esteem. Our education system focuses on marks and not much on personality development. So, young adults who emerge from prestigious universities often lack social skills. This is remedied through monitored social interactions and activities. But many of my clients are not satisfied with this approach and demand medication. While advertising for medicines is not allowed in India, many of these youths are consumers of American media. Hence, they are exposed to the ads of antidepressants promising instant relief. It is a huge effort to convince them otherwise. A few however resort to self-medication. Even with the government's diktat to chemists preventing sale of scheduled drugs without a valid prescription, there are many who sell them like OTC products. All the while, people with serious mental health issues refuse to take medications!'

'Disease mongering' refers to the practice of broadening or expanding the diagnostic boundaries of illnesses for profit. Pharmaceutical companies tend to aggressively promote their public awareness through various means. In the US, this may mean direct advertisements, while in other countries, it takes the form of articles, social media posts, indirect endorsements from opinion leaders, etc.

Way back in 1976, Henry Gadsden, CEO of Pharma major, Merck spoke about his dream to make drugs for healthy people, thus increasing the market size for Merck.[1] His dream is now a sad reality.

The opioid overdose crisis in the US can be attributed to disease mongering.[2] According to the CDC, 'from 1999 to 2018, more than 232,000 people died in the United States from overdoses involving prescription opioids.' The drug manufacturers not only tried to encourage unapproved uses of the opioids, they also tried to influence the community's perception about managing pain and addiction to painkillers. Some of the more intrepid marketers even introduced a new medical condition called 'pseudoaddiction'. The general idea of pseudoaddiction is that a patient treated with opioids who has symptoms of addiction or a withdrawal syndrome is not in fact addicted but in need of a stronger dose of opioids.

Meanwhile in India, painkiller addiction is on the increase. Many companies fearing lawsuits in the US are flooding Asian markets with these drugs. One such medicine, tramadol, a class of opioid easily available over the counter, is touted to be non-addictive. Many people, especially slum dwellers and manual workers, pop in these medications like candy. The Indian government took notice and announced a clampdown on the drug in 2018. Within months, a group of pain specialists from seven Southeast Asian countries, including three from influential hospitals in India, published a paper in the *Journal of Pain Research*. 'Tramadol: a Valuable Treatment for Pain in Southeast Asian Countries' made the case that 'the weak opioid tramadol has become the analgesic most frequently used in the region to treat moderate to severe pain.' The paper concluded: 'If it were to become a controlled substance, the standard of pain management in the region would decline.' The paper was funded by Grünenthal of Germany, a company that signed a deal in May 2018 to allow Mundipharma to market and distribute its tramadol product, Tramal, in China. Authors included pain specialists who have received consulting and lecturing fees from Pfizer, Johnson & Johnson and Mundipharma, a network of companies controlled by the Sackler family, owners of Connecticut-based Purdue Pharma.[3]

Vadodara-based gynaecologist Dr Vasudha Doshi* said to us, 'In the last five years or so, there has been a definite uptick in in the number of teenagers having sex. I am not worried about the moral aspect, but of the health of these girls. In the last week alone, I had three young girls saying that they not only engaged in sex, but their go-to contraceptive method was the morning-after pill. These pills are meant to be an emergency contraceptive and not a replacement for other methods. They are influenced by the ads they see on TV. I am not saying that these ads increase sexual promiscuity but I do feel that they tend to leave an impression on these young people and its excessive use may cause serious health concerns later.'

Pharma companies in India, by law, are not allowed to advertise directly to the consumer. Despite the law, pharma companies find enough loopholes. Indian consumers are being constantly exposed to advertisements for prescription as well as non-prescription medicines via television, internet, social media and other forms of media. Knowledge about pharmaceutical products obtained from various sources that are followed by the literate and illiterate person without consulting a pharmacist or physician leads to the practice of self-medication.[4]

Clinical Trials

Pradeep Gehlot, an autorickshaw driver from Indore, admitted his father Srikrishna Gehlot to a government hospital[5] after he complained of chest pain and breathlessness. His father was duly admitted, and Pradeep was asked to sign a few papers. These papers were in English (while the papers should have been in the local language) and Pradeep was told that the treatment would be free of cost and Srikrishna would be administered imported medicines. Little did they know that unknowingly, they had signed up for a clinical trial. Srikrishna's health deteriorated, and he died within two years of starting the trial. Pradeep shared his story with an NGO, which helped him lodge a complaint, following which the doctor's medical license was suspended for three months.

Pharma companies routinely conduct clinical trials—research that examines and studies the effect of new treatments and medications on humans. The Declaration of Helsinki states that 'Every clinical trial must be registered in a publicly accessible database before recruitment of the first subject.'[6] Volunteers who participate in the study must agree to the rules and terms outlined in the trial protocol. The trials are monitored by agencies as mandated by the country's government.[7] Researchers, doctors, all health professionals associated with this trial are expected to adhere to the rules set by these agencies. There is a lot of benefit to patients in trials. They get access to groundbreaking and lifesaving treatments they would not get access to otherwise.

One of the reasons India is a favourable market for clinical trials is the low cost for conducting them, compared to the Western world. Also, many potential participants would not have received treatment for the condition, and this helps in getting better data. India is also known for its hospital networks, professionals and research sites that meet global standards. Many of the clinical research firms are ethical and have strict volunteer-recruiting protocol, but there are quite a few that do not really bother about ethics.

> India is also known for a large number of people living below the poverty line who can become hapless guinea pigs in the name of 'research'. Some of the most shocking cases are:[7]
>
> - Unauthorized clinical trials of a vaccine against cervical cancer were conducted by an NGO on 25,000 minor girls in Khamman, Andhra Pradesh, and in Vadodara, Gujarat.
> - A government-funded hospital in Bhopal was conducting clinical trials on patients without their knowledge.
> - The MGM Medical College in Indore enrolled children into illegal drug tests for nearly ten years.

- At a government-run regional cancer centre in Thiruvananthapuram, twenty-five patients of oral cancer were given an experimental drug.
- Poor illiterate women from Guntur, Andhra Pradesh, were lured in for an illegal clinical trial for a breast cancer drug.

Be it orphanages, NGOs claiming to safeguard the rights of women or other organizations 'protecting' human rights—there are many unsavoury elements who coerce innocent people into these illegal trials. Some of them are promised money, while others are just forced into participation. There are brokers all around the country who source participants for trials. The innocent victims are rarely compensated fully and often pay with their lives.

In 2012, the NGO Swasthya Adhikar Manch filed a public interest petition on these illegal clinical trials. The Supreme Court came down heavily on the government and expressed shock at what it said was a 'disturbing' figure of 3,458 deaths and 14,320 serious side-effects documented among volunteers of clinical trials that were conducted in India between 2005 and 2012.[8]

What is worse is that out of all the drug trials that take place in India, around 40 per cent of the resulting medicines never reach the Indian market.[9]

The Supreme Court of India did call for more stringent regulations and closer monitoring of clinical trials. While the conditions may be a little better than what it was before 2013, illegal trials continue, and thousands of innocent Indian lives continue to be affected by corporate greed.

The Manufacturing Process

The pollution levels in the Edulabad Lake on the outskirts of Hyderabad has skyrocketed in the last decade.[10] In 2017, thousands of fish were washed ashore due to the toxic pollution. The residents of the village were also affected. The children attending the school near the lake developed skin and eye problems. A few children developed epilepsy. The skin issues are not limited to children. Adults who work in the paddy fields frequently develop skin rashes that do not heal with allopathic medicines. A local doctor opines that this may be due to the antibiotic resistance developed by the locals. Farmers have also noticed spontaneous abortions by their cows, a phenomenon that was unknown a few years ago.

Hyderabad is the centre of India's bulk drug manufacturing industry and pharmaceutical plants that manufacture active pharmaceutical ingredients (APIs) that are used to manufacture medicines. Unfortunately, Hyderabad is also the centre of pharmaceutical pollution.

A 2016 report[11] revealed high levels of drug-resistant bacteria in areas surrounding pharmaceutical factories in Hyderabad and Visakhapatnam, where a substantial share of the world's antibiotics is manufactured, as well as in New Delhi and Chennai. In total, out of thirty-four sites tested, sixteen were found to be harbouring bacteria resistant to antibiotics. At four of these sites, resistance to three major classes of antibiotics (cephalosporins, carbapenems and fluoroquinolones) was detected. Resistance to one or two of these classes of antibiotics were found at twelve more sites.

A recent study[12] by IIT Madras on pharmaceutical pollution in the Kaveri found anti-inflammatories like ibuprofen and diclofenac, antihypertensives such as atenolol and isoprenaline, enzyme inhibitors like perindopril, stimulants like caffeine, antidepressants such as carbamazepine, and antibiotics such as ciprofloxacin in the river that is the lifeline of lakhs of people.

Previous studies[13] by the IIT Delhi team reported the presence of several antibiotics, the most potent ones being found in Delhi's wastewater, and how such antibiotics are being transported to the Yamuna through the sewage system.

In a country with a myriad issues, pharmaceutical pollution tends to get swept under the rug. The pharma industry is one of the fastest growing industries and is a huge employment generator. India is seen as the hub for manufacturing generic drugs. Taking action against offenders would affect the production and economic development of the areas. Then, why would governments worry too much about pollution and how it affects you and me?

Questionable Practices

Chandigarh-based neurologist Dr Mona Chawla* is in a fix. 'There is a lot of pressure from all around to prescribe generic drugs instead of brand name drugs. I agree that the cost of a generic is much cheaper than a brand name drug. For example, Lyrica, which I frequently prescribe for neuropathic pain is priced at around ₹58 per capsule, while there are other Indian generics available at as low as ₹1.85 per capsule. That's such a wide gap. But in my experience, the efficacy of Lyrica is far superior to a generic. I am not saying that all brand names are superior, but in this case, Pfizer spent years developing this medicine and manufactures it under stringent quality conditions. Every step of the manufacturing process is important and if a company adheres to the process, in my opinion, there is no way that there can be such a vast difference in the price. How do I, then, with a clear conscience, prescribe a generic? And remember, all generics are not equal. If I just write the generic name, the chemist is free to sell whatever gives them the highest profitability. At the end, the patient suffers.'

India is known as the 'pharmacy to the world' mainly because of its cost-effective production and the sheer size of the market. The Indian pharmaceutical industry is currently valued at around $50 billion and is expected to grow at a compound annual growth rate of 10.7 per cent by 2030. The pharmaceutical market in India is expected to reach $65 billion by 2024, and $130 billion by 2030.[14] India's pharmaceuticals industry is the third largest by volume and the thirteenth largest by value in the world, producing more than 60,000 generic drugs across sixty therapeutic categories.[15] A generic drug is a medication created to be the same as an existing approved brand name drug in dosage form, safety, strength, route of administration, quality and performance characteristics.[16]

All new drugs are protected by patent for a period of time. This helps the company that worked on and launched the drug to recover the money that was spent on years of research, or the money spent on buying the rights to the drug. Under patent laws, other companies cannot sell a similar drug. Once the patent expires, other companies can develop the drug and market it. These drugs are called 'generic medicines'. These generics will differ from brand names in shape, size, colour and packaging, or may contain inactive ingredients that do not contribute to the treatment effect of the drug.

In the earlier days, drugs were covered by a patent that protected the end product only. If you manufactured the same drug using a slightly different process, then you were in the clear. So, many Indian pharma companies tweaked one small step in the process and launched copycat drugs without investing anything at all in research and development (R&D). With the shift from a product patent to a process patent system, copying became much more difficult.

This change from product patent to process patent meant that the Indian pharma industry had to quickly invest in R&D, at least for form's sake. They did so to some extent but, even today, Indian pharma is known more for bulk drug manufacturing and production of lower cost equivalents rather than pathbreaking discoveries. There are many concerns related to the generic drugs manufactured in India. Often, it has been found that these drugs contain less than the required amount of APIs. The manufacturing conditions in many plants—characterized by poor levels of quality control, poor process control, non-adherence to good manufacturing practices (GMPs)—are questionable. Every year, we see instances of how Indian pharma companies were found to have violated GMP norms by fudging data or cutting corners. In 2022, there were reports of seventy children in The Gambia dying, allegedly after consuming a made-in-India cough syrup. Later, there were reports of eighteen children dying in Uzbekistan after ingesting a cough syrup manufactured in India. Between May 2022 and January 2023, the CDC in the US reported that a certain brand of eyedrops manufactured in India may have been involved in infecting fifty-five people across twelve US states and causing one death. The WHO red-flagged as many as seven Indian manufactured cough syrups and the investigation is ongoing.[17]

The US Food and Drug Administration (FDA) quite often sends warning letters to Indian pharma companies for repeatedly fudging data and short-circuiting clinical trials. Mind you, these are not small, fly-by-night companies but big names in India, including some listed on the stock exchange. To be fair, data fudging is a global problem in the pharma industry and not restricted to India alone, but the laxity in regulations and corruption makes it rampant in India.

India's Central Drugs Standard Control Organization (CDSCO) does not make its testing data on drugs publicly available. This is a huge issue as it leaves consumers clueless about the quality and efficacy of the drugs that they are consuming.

India is one of the global leaders in the manufacturing of fixed-dose combinations (FDCs), combinations of more than one generic drug. Well-known pharma industry whistleblower, ex-Ranbaxy employee and author of *Bottle of Lies* Dinesh Thakur comments:

> FDC, to be frank, is non-sense according to me. While the CDSCO issues approval for FDCs, it is the state FDA, which gives permission for manufacturing and marketing. Due to this liberal licensing system, we have large number of FDCs whose efficacy, safety and rationality is questionable. Majority of these FDCs are formulated with marketing as primary interest and add no value to its therapeutic usage.[18]

India boasts of a network of around 3,000 drug companies and 10,500 manufacturing units.[19] But how many of these comply to world class quality standards is anybody's guess.

The Pharma-Doctor Nexus

Around a decade back, a medical representative (MR) was in my consultation room. He was in the middle of explaining a new drug that had been launched by his company when he got a call. He sought my permission to take the call as he said it was important. I could hear a high-pitched voice from the other side and the MR uttered some apologies in a conciliatory tone. Finally, as he hung up after a few minutes, the MR gave me a hapless look. Out of politeness, I enquired if all was well. The words tumbled out of his mouth, 'That was a doctor—very senior and very well respected. As part of our sales promotion, we are sponsoring an overseas conference for him. As is our norm, we booked him in business class. After a few days, the doctor called me asking me to book a ticket for his wife too. I tried telling him that it is not part of the company policy, but he was insistent. I spoke to my boss, and we got the necessary approvals from the management and booked a ticket for the doctor's wife. Now he is upset that her ticket has not been booked in business class. Over the call, he was threatening to stop prescribing our company's medicines if we do not upgrade her. Imagine the utter shamelessness! The difference in the cost of the tickets is what he earns on a few patient consultations! Now, I have to go back to my boss with this request and I am sure to get a talking-to from him. I should have never joined this field!' he ended with a sigh.

My friends in the pharma industry tell me that this is far from being an unusual case. Doctors often keep track of their prescriptions and have a good idea of the revenue they generate for the company. Hence, they feel entitled to demand their pound of flesh. So what if it is illegal?

Drug discovery and development is a long, costly and high-risk process that takes over ten to fifteen years with an average cost of over $1–2 billion for each new drug to be approved for clinical use. The failure rate in drug discovery is very high, as much as 90 per cent.[20] Clearly, the stakes are very high for pharma companies, and to offset this failure rate, they need to maximize revenues on the drugs that finally make it to the market. Hence, the need for aggressive marketing. Since direct advertising to the consumer is banned in India, the companies must market to the doctors and chemists. In a cutthroat business environment, the companies vie with each other to come up with promotions that will ensure that doctors prescribe their company's drugs.

The nexus between pharma and the medical industry is deep and all-encompassing. For us, the doctor receiving air tickets for a junket abroad may be the visible end of the spectrum but at every level—from drug discovery to drug validation, interactions with drug control authorities, advisory boards, clinical trials and retail sales—the hold of pharma over doctors and chemists is strong and continuous.

The unholy link between the pharma industry and doctors is a global one, but in India little attempt has been made to regulate the practices that lead to corruption.

As I mentioned earlier, pharma companies need to look at aggressive marketing tactics to make profits. While companies may have a basket of products, they rely on a handful of 'blockbuster' drugs to maximize revenues. In India, there are two points of persuasion. The first is the prescribing doctor and the second is the dispensing chemist. A 2016 report[21] on dispensing practices in the IT capital of India, Bengaluru, puts the percentage of dispensing by chemists without prescriptions at almost 45 per cent. Across the country, chemists regularly dispense all categories of medicines—be it analgesics, antibiotics, antipsychotic medicines, sleeping tablets, etc.—without prescription. Often, chemists can persuade the customer to buy another brand of the same combination. The reasons can be 'no stock', 'this brand is better', 'this brand is cheaper', etc. Pharma companies in India target both these segments to increase sales of their products.

The sight of formally dressed representatives in the waiting rooms of doctors is a common sight. They wait for hours on end to meet the doctor and 'persuade' them to dispense their company's products. Gone are the days when doctors were gifted pens, calendars, diaries, etc., by the companies as freebies. Today, the cost of the freebies paid by pharma companies in India is estimated to be ₹4,000 crores annually![22]

As I have mentioned time and again in this book, contrary to popular opinion, all doctors are not rolling in money, and they have similar financial concerns as everyone else and are not averse to freebies. I reiterate that I am not painting all doctors in India with the same brush but highlighting the bad practices that need to be made public.

Samuel Oomen,* a retired pharma salesman, shared some vignettes from his experience. 'We used to have frequent sales training where medical representatives (MRs) with the best sales records would share their success stories and strategies. One such story came from an MR who managed two small towns in a district. He organized a conference in a five-star property in the nearest city for around fifteen doctors from both towns. He ensured that the invite was extended to spouses too. After an hour of obligatory medical discussions, the doctors were free to socialize and enjoy the five-star amenities. The lavish dinner included liquor, where quite a few doctors got sozzled. The doctors thoroughly enjoyed the two-day break, and soon, were only prescribing our brands. All of us copied this strategy and as a region, we clocked the highest sales for that year!' Reminiscing further, he added, 'Of course, this did not last. Our competitor raised the bar and took the doctors to Dubai for a "conference". We responded by taking the doctors to Turkey. Soon, it became the norm rather than the exception and doctors demanded more and more from us—business class tickets, tickets for spouse, suites in hotels instead of rooms. There is no end to greed!' he concluded.

Pharma companies are the major sponsors of most medical conferences in India, where leading doctors, who are speakers at these events, often promote individual brands for a fee. These companies also set up advisory boards for individual drugs and recruit specialist doctors to them. The board meetings are held periodically, often at exotic locales, making it an all-expense paid trip for the doctors. This is over and above the remuneration they receive for serving as a board member!

Touching upon the area of training, Oomen shared, 'When I joined the industry almost thirty years back, training was focused on product knowledge. But over the years, trainings are focused on how to manage doctors. Today, an MR may not even know about all the aspects of the drug they are promoting but will know what carrot to dangle to which doctor.' Shaking his head, he continues, 'It is a reflection of today's times that bribes are not just limited to international trips, electrical appliances, gadgets, etc., but also include women! Can you imagine how demeaning it is for us salespeople?'

A report on pharmaceutical marketing practices echoing these points was released by a public health group, Support for Advocacy and Training to Health initiatives (SATHI)[23]. The report caused an outcry in the community but only because it accused pharma companies of supplying women to doctors. The rest was mostly taken as a given.

'Our sales were not limited to selling to doctors,' continued Oomen. 'One of us realized that we could use their wives to influence their decisions. So, we would collect coupons from neighbourhood supermarkets and deliver them to the doctors' households. Higher the value of the doctor for us, higher the value of the coupon. We would ensure that their wives knew which company was sponsoring the coupons and which drug needs to be prescribed by their husbands.'

Other companies caught on and soon, fuel coupons, e-wallets, credit cards, etc., were given as freebies. Companies also purchased cars or two-wheelers for doctors and paid the EMIs on their behalf. This ensured the doctors' commitment to their brands—at least until the EMI was paid off!

'Do not for a moment think that women doctors are less susceptible to bribes,' said Oomen. 'Of course, we had to deal with women doctors in a slightly different manner. The whole operation has to be more subtle, never aggressive or overt. A few doctors may need to be cajoled, but at the end, we manage to break them. In fact, it used to be a headache sometimes as women doctors are generally much more meticulous when it comes to maintaining accounts and they would demand their pound of flesh with exacting detail.'

Another industry veteran, Ajinkya Deodhar,* shared his experience with us, 'I made an analysis of how these freebies evolved over the years. Of course, these are from my experience and from discussions with colleagues, but I would think that this is a fairly accurate summary. In the 1980s, MRs would generally give booklets about the medicine or the condition. We would pay a few doctors to write these booklets. We also started gifting customized products like, say, a couch, or a delivery table for their clinics. For doctors who were setting up a nursing home with an attached pharmacy, we would pass on heavy discounts to the pharmacy. With the 90s, our focus shifted to creating awareness about screening centres—whether it was diabetes or other diseases. We set up these centres for doctors. In return, they were expected to prescribe our drugs. We also started supplying IT support through patient database support systems. Remember, technology was not as prevalent in those days! The turn of the century saw increased competition in the industry, so we went all out with the freebies. Be it honoraria for certain advisory positions, international speaking assignments, high-profile conferences, referral fees, inducements for Phase 3 clinical trials, sponsored research papers showing our drugs in a good light or heavily subsidized loans—the list is endless.'

When we asked if they were not worried about legal ramifications, Deodhar said, 'There is no law, merely suggestions, to not indulge in such practices. And yes, companies have their own code of ethics, which we bypass by using middlemen or brokers instead of doing it ourselves. It is all about achieving our sales numbers, not how we achieve them!'

Other industry insiders I interviewed concur that in the early days the trend was more towards giving doctors gifts, which gradually became more and more expensive. Then the demand was for money and pharma companies shifted to handing out cash. The sums today are way above what can be given in cash. So almost all companies write out cheques. Doctors possibly write off these amounts as professional income in their tax returns.

Spandana Girish* is a marketing specialist for one of India's leading pharma companies. Among her other responsibilities, she manages conferences and organizes public speaking events. In an interview with me, she said, 'Medical events are now big in India. The speakers' fees have touched the roof. Specialists and high-profile doctors charge almost ₹2 lakh per hour as their fees. No self-respecting doctor would accept anything less than ₹25,000 for speaking at an event nowadays. Hospitals, big and small, are savvy enough to use us to sponsor their exhibitions. The hospitals earn monies from stalls, participants, etc., while we—the companies—bear all the expenses.'

If the pharma industry is neck deep in kickbacks, the medical devices industry is perhaps submerged in it. Multiple industry sources tell me that it is extremely rare to find a hospital or an orthopaedic surgeon in India who does not get a cut from the implants they place inside patients' bodies. Hospitals and surgeons get kickbacks of 15–20 per cent of the price charged on the implant.

Industry insiders say that there are some specialities that are worse than others. Diabetes with its massive patient population and expensive insulin, oncology and rheumatology with their extremely high-cost newer generation biological drugs and cardiology with its long-term care needs are specialties where the nexus is deep.

Deodhar reserves his choicest remarks for the doctors who demand that the companies give them money to build hospitals. 'It is not a small sum of money. The monies are given upfront, and we generally use a middleman for the transaction as the company records must be clean. Doctors pay us back by writing prescriptions of our brands, pushing our drugs and devices for the stipulated number of years. Some of the staff in the hospitals are in on the take and often cut their deals with pharma and device manufacturers behind the backs of their management. If you think that the government sector is corrupt, you haven't met scheming doctors and purchase managers of private hospitals,' he seethed.

Doctors and a social conscience go hand in hand. Not always though. Fatima Zahir,* a corporate social responsibility (CSR) consultant, says, 'Do you know that pharma companies set up foundations or NGOs in the names of the doctors and hospitals? The companies pump in monies as grants or donations, treating these as their CSR contribution, while the doctors and hospitals can use the monies as they please.'

As I mentioned earlier, the kickbacks are not restricted to doctors and hospitals only. Pharmacists around the country receive their share of bribes too. This can be in the form of helmets for the employees to a vehicle for the owner. They are also given heavier discounts and schemes to promote a certain drug. Unlike in more developed countries, there is no central agency monitoring the dispensing of medicines. Elizabeth Richards, a sixty-five-year-old homemaker, says, 'I lived for nearly two decades outside India before returning to my hometown of Pune. I am under treatment for fibromyalgia and my medications include Duloxetine, Pregabalin and Tramadol. When I was in Dubai, I could refill my prescription only after a doctor's consult. Even there, I needed to give my original ID card every time. These medicines fall under the controlled drugs list, and I would not be given a prescription of more than sixty tablets at a time, at the maximum. But here, I just send the list to my local chemist and these medicines are home delivered. I have never been asked for a prescription. I can order any quantity I want!' While it may be easier for Elizabeth, dispensing these medicines without prescriptions can lead to adverse effects on the patient. It is also easier for addicts to buy the medicines and get their fix.

Some marketing techniques tend to backfire. Oomen shared, 'A few years back, one of the companies came up with a scheme of buying cars for the doctors. The pharma company was to pay an upfront amount and the EMIs for a fixed period. The remaining amount was to be paid by the doctors themselves. So far, so good! The problem started when a few doctors missed out on the EMIs, and the banks/finance companies resorted to seizing the cars back. How? Simple, they hired some goons who would show up anywhere, eject the doctor (or whoever was in the car) and drive away with the car. Obviously, the doctors were not happy with this. Their reputation was at stake. They promptly turned against the company and threatened them with dire consequences if the matter was not resolved. The company ended up forking out much more than what was planned and cleared the payments. Not only that, but they also ended up antagonizing the very doctors they wanted to win over!'

Lest I leave you with the impression that all doctors are corrupt, let me assure you that there are many doctors who are highly ethical and say no to kickbacks. Deodhar shared this story of a doctor in a small town in Maharashtra: 'The doctor refused to accept any bribes or a cut from the sales. He asked for a lot of samples and instead of selling them, he actually distributed the medicines to the poor. He demanded that we conduct free health camps. In my experience, doctors from small clinics have higher levels of integrity, even if they are not raking in the money, while superspecialists from upmarket hospitals often make mind-boggling demands.'

How does all this affect you? Well, a medicine is supposed to help and not create any problem. And it should be prescribed only when you need it, not when the doctor needs it. How can one rely on doctors who prescribe not with the patient's best interests, but with their wallet in mind? And there is no way for a layperson to figure out which doctor is taking a kickback and which one is not. The kickback industry significantly increases the cost of healthcare as well as the risks for the patient. There are no studies that reveal how much extra a patient ends up paying because of this nexus. But in a country where still over 60 per cent of the healthcare cost is borne out of pocket, any increase is too big a burden to bear.

Toothless Regulations

Why has the law not been made stringent enough to enable a crackdown on such corrupt practices? After much delay, the Government of India came out with the Uniform Code of Pharmaceuticals Marketing Practices (UCPMP) in 2015. This, however, is voluntary and so has virtually no teeth. Violations will be reported to the pharmaceutical associations themselves for action.

In March 2022, the government issued a draft Uniform Code for Medical Devices Marketing Practices (UCMDMP). Like the UCPMP, this draft is also a voluntary code and, so, no one truly cares much for it. Medical device procurement is another area where corruption is rampant in the government and private sectors. Very little has been done to regulate it.

On 2 August 2023, the National Medical Council (NMC) put out a set of guidelines in an attempt to regulate the enormous influence that the pharma industry wields over doctors in India. The NMC said individual doctors should not accept sponsorships in any form from the pharma industry and that violation could lead to their license being suspended for up to three months. In effect, the pharma industry could no longer sponsor doctors to attend medical conferences in India or abroad or take care of their expenses during such trips. Any sponsorship of medical conferences by the pharma industry had to be done through medical associations.

This rule has existed in most parts of the developed world for several years and was much needed in India. The US, for instance, has the Physician Payments Sunshine Act, 2010, which requires full disclosure of payments to doctors, hospitals and other healthcare service providers so that the general public can judge for itself if doctors are being influenced to prescribe particular medicines.[24]

The announcement in India, however, led to an outrage from the medical community. The directive also specified that doctors must prescribe generic drugs and not brand names, which is not entirely a practical or wise decision. Doctors across the country latched on to this issue and tried to derail the entire notification.

It was not long before they were successful. On 23 August, in less than three weeks, the entire notification was put on hold, effectively ending yet another attempt to break the nexus between the industry and doctors.

The reason for the failure is simple: a lack of political will. Health is not an election issue in India, and visible spending on hospitals and healthcare facilities is all that matters. Irrespective of political affiliations, no government is willing to bell this cat. After the recent cough syrup fatalities, there is increased international clamour and some countries are even threatening to ban Indian products.

The unanimous opinion across the industry is that only the government, through stringent regulation, punitive fines, cancellation of licenses and even the threat of imprisonment, can remedy the situation. The situation is way past any self-regulation by the industry or by medical associations.

Some pharma company bosses have concerns with the manner in which their industry functions. One of them told me that to survive in the Indian market, they had simply no choice but to keep the payoffs to doctors and chemists going. 'In a market where every competitor is following a practice, it becomes virtually impossible to swim against the tide. So, we have to go along. To ease our conscience, we do a fair amount of CSR, fund free health camps, etc.'

The UCPMP was expected to have at least some impact but being a voluntary code, it has had almost none. Doctors who conduct clinical trials can make a killing (pardon the pun) from the pharma company. Having been on an ethical committee for the sanctioning of clinical trials, I can vouch for the fact that it was a massive challenge to ensure that the conduct of the trial was not vitiated or corrupted by the company sponsoring the trial.

The 'Pharmacy to the World' needs a major house cleaning and a strong regulatory system to ensure that the medicines it produces heal, or at the very least do not harm the consumer.

What Do We Do about It?

It is my considered opinion that the government needs to reintroduce the rules it had proposed in August 2023, which it has put on hold. I agree that there will be challenges and it may delay some genuine academic activities. But isn't this better than continuing with a rotten system? The industry will adapt to the new normal if the government enforces the notification.

That will be a good starting point. If the Government sticks to its guns, then over a period of several months, the industry will adapt. Pharma companies may start sponsoring medical associations to hold events. While that too has its drawbacks, it would be a whole lot better than the present system.

It is imperative that the CDSCO publishes data on the efficacy of all drugs and the testing it does in the public domain. This will give people more knowledge about the shenanigans that some pharma players may indulge in. The greater scrutiny will ensure increased adherence to the rules.

Clinical trials must be regulated even more tightly. This is one area where there have been some improvements over the last decade but there are still too many loopholes that exploit the ignorance of patients. Clinical trials are an important part of drug development and must be conducted in an ethical and legal manner.

Manufacturing practices must come under heavy scrutiny to ensure quality of the end products, prevent water and soil pollution, and overall guarantee that the pill that is finally swallowed by the patient does not cause harm.

Both doctors and pharma companies must be punished if they are involved in prescriptions for payments. Chemists must not be allowed to sell prescription drugs as OTC medication.

Finally, the public must start to learn and care more about putting an end to the pernicious practices of Big Pharma.

A policymaker who had worked with the government on pharma regulation in the early 2000s told me that public pressure is the key to get the government to act and ensure better regulation. We, as, the public need to demand for change.

> The National Medical Commission (NMC) has issued comprehensive guidelines for the professional conduct of registered doctors in India under The NMC Registered Medical Practitioner (Professional Conduct) Regulations 2023. This was later withdrawn.
>
> Some key points from the guidelines included:
>
> | Aspect | Guidelines |
> |---|---|
> | Use of Social Media | Doctors can use social media for providing information or announcements. The information must be verifiable and not misleading. The guideline warns against soliciting patients through social media. Prohibited: discussing specifics of patient treatment and sharing patient scans online. Patient privacy must be maintained. Advised to follow decorum when interacting online. |

Aspect	Guidelines
Prescription Practices	Doctors required to prescribe generic medicines. Exceptions for cases requiring specific brand names due to narrow therapeutic index or exceptional situations. Encouraged to educate patients about the equivalence of generic and branded medicines.
Right to Refuse Treatment	Doctors have the right to refuse treatment for abusive, unruly or violent patients and relatives. Must not refuse treatment in medical emergencies. Prohibited from discrimination based on various grounds.
Continuous Professional Development	Doctors mandated to undergo continuous learning throughout active years. Accumulate thirty credit points in relevant fields every five years. Annual sessions of at least three credits (ideally six). No more than 50 per cent of training should be conducted online.

Aspect	Guidelines
Professional Conduct	Doctors are prohibited from participating in conferences and CPD sessions sponsored by pharmaceutical companies. Each doctor shall display the unique registration ID assigned to them in prescriptions, certificates and money receipts given to patients. Doctors cannot be involved in fee splitting, earning commissions from diagnostic services, endorsing a product or person, operating an open-to-all medical store, etc. Prohibited from receiving gifts, hospitality or monetary benefits from pharmaceutical companies, medical device companies or corporate hospitals.
Disciplinary action	Five levels of disciplinary actions, ranging from warning to permanent debarment from practice for Registered Medical Practitioner.

9
Are More Hospitals and Doctors Really the Solution?

Suresh Gopal* is a fifty-two-year-old banking professional who migrated to the US around fifteen years ago. His father, Gopal,* a widower, chose to stay back in Chennai, in spite of Suresh's best efforts to get him to move to Chicago. Resigned to his father's decision, Suresh would fly down to Chennai every year and spend some time with his father. During his stay, he would take his father for various medical checkups. His father was diabetic and hypertensive, and had undergone a coronary angioplasty in 2003. 'My father was healthy, despite all his conditions,' said Suresh. 'He had an active life, and despite not having his family around, he was surrounded by friends and hence was not lonely. All this changed during the pandemic. He was boxed inside his home and had little social connect. Also, his regular medical checkups could not happen due to all the travel and commuting restrictions. Around September 2022, he developed rectal bleeding and was rushed to the hospital by friends. He was initially diagnosed with a bleeding polyp in his intestines and doctors recommended that he stay in the hospital, given his age and other health issues, until it had been dealt with. Given the situation, the family and the patient agreed. Over the next few weeks, doctors kept recommending different treatments and we kept complying with the recommendations. My father, however, did not become better. In fact, he got a lot worse. He pleaded with me to take him home and let him die at home. But I was too scared to take the risk. It was around the fourth week when one of the attending doctors broke the news that my father was resistant to all antibiotics, and nothing could be really done. In addition, he had picked up a urinary tract infection (UTI) during one of his stays in the ICU. It was just wait and watch and I watched as my father faded into an agonizing death. While I agree that no one is immortal, I am wracked with guilt over the pain and sheer agony that my father had to endure in his last few weeks. This guilt is compounded as I am not sure if admitting him to the hospital for that long a period was the right choice. He finally died because of the infection he picked up in the hospital and not because of any pre-existing disease.'

Suresh's story is not really unique. It is an open secret that hospital acquired infections (HAIs) are more common in India than in the Western world. HAIs are acquired by a patient during the process of care (including preventive, diagnostic and treatment services) in a hospital or other healthcare facility. These infections can also appear after discharge. They may also be acquired by health workers during healthcare delivery and by visitors.

Even before the coronavirus pandemic, there was a high rate of HAIs. Unfortunately, precise numbers aren't available as hospitals tend to fudge data or not maintain records of this at all.

When we think of solutions for better healthcare, the obvious answers include more healthcare providers and, of course, more hospitals. But is this really the solution? There has been a considerable increase in the number of hospitals in the last decade or so but where is the growth happening? There is also an increase in the number of medical training centres, but what is the quality of the graduates from these facilities? Has anyone done a cost–benefit analysis for this strategy?

These are questions that need to be answered.

Hospitals in India

As a friend said, 'A business in education or health rarely fails!' Look around where you live. Have you noticed a spurt in the number of educational institutions and hospitals? Especially if you live in a metro city, chances are there would be a hospital within a radius of 5 kms! It is likely that it is a part of a larger corporate chain. It is also possible that you may not really find too many single practitioner setups in your locality.

Healthcare is one of the fastest growing industries in India. Since 2016, it has been growing at a compound annual growth rate of 22 per cent. It has become one of the largest sectors of revenue and employment generation.[1]

The hospital industry in India accounted for 70 per cent of the total healthcare market in the 2021 financial year. Hospitals include PHCs, district hospitals and general hospitals, and top and mid-tier private hospitals and nursing homes. The hospital infrastructure industry is expected to grow with both domestic and foreign players entering this market. In fact, this is one of the few industries that allows 100 per cent foreign direct investment (FDI). Between 2000 to 2020, the FDI in health infrastructure has been an eye-watering ₹55.6 thousand crores.[2] The initial public offerings (IPOs) of Dr Lal PathLabs, HealthCare Global (HCG), Narayana Health and Thyrocare were oversubscribed—a clear demonstration of investor confidence in this sector.

The growth is not just limited to metros but extends to Tier-II and Tier-III cities. Sixty-five per cent of the available hospital beds cater to around 50 per cent of the population concentrated in the states of Uttar Pradesh, Maharashtra, Karnataka, Tamil Nadu, Telangana, West Bengal and Kerala.[3] Obviously, the other 50 per cent of the population living in the rest of the twenty-one states and eight union territories have access only to 35 per cent of the beds. Investors are not blind to this huge potential and neither is the government, which aims to ensure equitable distribution for all citizens in all parts of the country.

The healthcare industry is the fourth largest employer in the country, contributing to around 10.4 per cent of total employment.[4] This translates to approximately 57.6 lakh jobs. While exact figures aren't available for the hospital industry, it would be fair to assume that at least 60–70 per cent of healthcare jobs are in this sector.

India has 1 bed for 1,000 people as against the WHO guidelines of 3 beds for every 1,000. As we know, this distribution is heavily skewed towards Tier-I and Tier-II cities and to a few states of the country.

In 1972, India had only 98 medical colleges. By 1981, there were 109 and by 1992 there were 128 across the country. By 2001, there were 189 colleges and 314 by 2011. Between 2011 and 2021, this number almost doubled to 595, out of which 302 are government medical colleges and 293 are private.[5]

The southern states (Andhra Pradesh, Karnataka, Telangana, Kerala, Tamil Nadu and Pondicherry) account for 20 per cent of India's population and has around 41 per cent of the medical seats, whereas the two most populous states of Uttar Pradesh and Bihar have only 11 per cent of the total.

The central and state governments are working towards increasing the number of medical colleges and the number of MBBS seats. There is also a focus on more equitable distribution of the seats across the country. The budgeted expenditure on the health sector reached 2.2 per cent of gross domestic product (GDP) in the 2022 financial year against 1.6 per cent in 2021.[6]

Excellent work indeed! This kind of effort and investment in this area is unprecedented. It also doesn't hurt that hospitals and medical colleges are potential vote pullers. Structures are visible and are proof that local politicians have worked for their constituency.

More hospitals are good, and more doctors are the need of the hour. Right? Not necessarily.

More Hospitals Are Not Always the 'Need of the Hour'

Innovations in the medical field are changing not only how hospitals are structured, but also how healthcare is delivered. More hospitals, more doctors and more paramedical staff are touted as the panacea for most of the disparities in healthcare access. Governments in India build hospitals and political parties in election manifestoes often promise more health centres. The assumption in the public mind is also that more hospitals mean better healthcare.

Let us examine this assumption to see if it is really true.

Clinical and surgical advancements

In recent years, clinical knowledge has seen a rapid advancement. Emergence of better drugs has meant that fewer patients with infectious diseases need hospitalization.

In the past, a diagnosis of HIV/AIDS was akin to a death sentence. But today, it has become more of a chronic condition in a significant number of patients. The development of newer antiviral medicines has changed the lives of many patients of hepatitis C. The increasing use of monoclonal antibodies and gene therapy means that drug therapies are quite effective in many conditions, and the need for invasive procedures has reduced. While we do have some distance to go before these therapies become affordable across the population, they are generally reducing the need for hospitalization.

Advancements in surgical procedures has led to shorter hospital stays. When a friend of mine went in for a joint replacement surgery around 2009, he stayed in the hospital for nearly a week. This is in sharp contrast with another friend who, after a similar procedure in 2022, was discharged within forty-eight hours.

The ease of administration of IV medication at home has also reduced the need for hospital stays.

More and more elective surgical procedures are now being performed as day-care procedures or surgeries thus obviating the need for overnight hospital stay (when a patient does not need to stay overnight in a hospital). Even a few decades earlier, it was necessary for patients who have undergone gall bladder removal to stay in the hospital for a few days. Pre- and post-operative care were essential parts of the procedure. But today, the patient comes to the hospital in the morning and leaves by evening, thereby eliminating the need for any overnight stay. Similarly, other procedures like appendicectomy, inguinal hernia repair, haemorrhoidectomy and hysterectomy are all now day-care procedures. In fact, in some specialties like ophthalmology, there is now virtually no need for hospitals, only for day-care clinics.

In many countries, coronary angioplasty is performed as a day-care procedure, and it will not be long before this trend comes to India too.

Technological advancements

A surgeon colleague of mine tells me that most of general surgery is now day-care. Some surgeries have been replaced altogether by procedures performed by other specialists like intervention radiologists. Use of advanced laparoscopic techniques and surgical robots have helped perform precision surgery, requiring a shorter hospital stay.

Some of us would have had experiences with remote consulting during the pandemic. This trend has not shown any signs of coming down, even after the world opened up. The convenience of consulting with a doctor without having to endure commuting hassles and waiting in the reception has quickly caught on. Most hospitals offer the choice of either in-person or video consults. Hospitals have also built their own platforms, thus ensuring patient confidentiality. Durga Jain* is a thirty-two-year-old busy executive and a mother of two. She says, 'I continue to work from home and my two children come home with the usual litany of childhood complaints. I find it so much easier to consult the doctor online. Earlier, it was such a hassle. Their illness would invariably coincide with some important work meeting. My husband and I would have to really stretch ourselves to take our child to the hospital. It meant taking the whole day off. It is so much easier now. I need to take out only twenty odd minutes from my workday. Even if the doctor suggests some bloodwork or similar tests, I can get it done from home. And the best part is that I am not paying extra for this service. I wish I could get my teen's braces done from the comfort of home! That's true over expectation,' she concludes with a laugh.

While remote braces may not yet be possible, a range of clinical services has and will continue to shift to remote modalities. I am sure that by 2030, there will be many more revolutionary changes.

Technology helps us monitor hypertension, diabetes and certain heart related concerns without the need for a physical visit. These measurements can be directly uploaded to an electronic health record. This helps patients to connect to specialists directly and get an early-stage intervention.

For example, Aravind Eye Hospitals and Sankara Nethralaya use telemedicine to serve patients in villages. They have set up IT-enabled vision centres and mobile vision clinics, linked to the main hospitals. This system has reduced the need for a physical hospital in villages, while at same time ensuring low-cost, high-quality medical service to a population which would otherwise have been underserved.

Technology also helps in cross-consultation, and the medical community can reach out to colleagues from different locations or specializations. Medical records can be shared by a click of a button and the patient benefits from the whole process.

An epidemic of lifestyle diseases

I was talking to a much older colleague and the conversation veered to the way his practice has changed over the years. In the course of the discussion, he commented, 'When

I started my practice almost four decades back, the scenario was so different. I used to have patients coming in with infections—mainly diarrhoea, TB and other chest infections. Cholera used to pop up quite frequently, as did typhoid. I am retired now but still see a few patients and have younger colleagues asking for my opinion. Today, it is more about hypertension, diabetes, heart issues, autoimmune conditions, chronic allergies, etc. Maybe it is the lifestyle changes, maybe it is the pollution or the food we eat. I also see more cases of obesity, even in the villages.'

We are witnessing a rapid epidemiological transition in India: there is a shift towards chronic non-communicable diseases along with socio-economic development. India is also the diabetic capital of the world with 7.7 crore diagnoses, and it is projected to increase to 13.4 crore by 2045. Non-communicable or chronic diseases account for 53 per cent of all deaths in India and 44 per cent of disability-adjusted life-years lost.[7] One of the biggest causes of early deaths in India is cardiovascular disease, which also contributes to one-fourth of all deaths in India. The population with hypertension is also steeply increasing across the country and is no longer limited to the urban population.

All this means that the way doctors practise medicine has also changed. Now, their job is as much counselling as prescribing medications. Ernakulam based endocrinologist Dr Mathew Chandy* says, 'Once the diagnosis of diabetes is established, it is then time for counselling. I have to repeat the same instructions over and over—on diet, exercise, sleep, hygiene, taking medications on time, monitoring, etc.

I tried printing out the advice and handing it to the patients but most of them still prefer to talk to me. I would be exhausted and felt that I wasn't giving enough time to the patients I meet later in the day. I finally hired and trained a nurse practitioner to answer all the questions, freeing me to meet more patients and concentrate on my work. My nurse practitioner also counsels the family of the patients and conducts all kinds of workshops on exercises, recipes, etc. Patients have seen the benefit and there are a few who prefer talking to her than to me! I am there only to look at the medical aspect.'

Mathew is not the only one who has done this. Dr Padmaja Rawandale,* a cardiologist in Nashik, comments, 'With all the advancements in cardiac care, more patients are surviving heart attacks and strokes. The time they spend at hospitals is reducing but, post-discharge, they need a lot of help to manage their day-to-day activities.'

Many doctors have trained nurses to counsel the patients. Most chronic patients take control of their health in a few years but need reassurance from an expert. After a certain point, the medications are also stable unless they have a flareup. The counselling can be either one-on-one or through support groups. Dr Humeira Badsha believes strongly in the power of support groups. She conducts regular patient outreach workshops and discusses the challenges of living with arthritis and teaches self-management techniques. Most of these workshops are conducted by experts in the field or by patient advocates.

This is better done in community settings with the focus being on prevention. Nagesh Dhar,* an entrepreneur who runs an agency that provides trained bedside assistants, says, 'My father was admitted into a hospital after a stroke. I am grateful to the medical team for their quick response and for ensuring that he survived. However, he was not discharged for almost fourteen days from the hospital as he needed to be monitored. It didn't help that he is diabetic. After the initial few days, my family found it difficult to manage my father. He hated the hospital setting and kept abusing us for not taking him back home. He is generally a placid person but now he would yell at us or plead with us. He lost interest in watching his favourite series and became listless. I was worried and did a bit of research on managing the situation. It was then that I found out that there was a lot of evidence that elderly patients lost a significant percent of muscle strength during hospitalization. It would be a formidable task for the patients to return to their pre-hospitalization health. I did in-depth research across the country and my team spoke to many doctors across specializations and geographies. Almost 90 per cent of the respondents agreed that the length of stay in a hospital can and should be reduced, provided that adequate care can be given at home. Better home monitoring technologies have become available, thus eliminating the need for a significant number of patients to be kept in hospital only to be monitored.

'Telemedicine has also emerged as a mainstream method of doctor consultation, further reducing the need for hospital stay and even outpatient follow-up visits. That was the seed for my venture. My company provides trained bedside assistants who can monitor the patients at the comfort of their home. This is also cheaper than hospitalization and frees up the time of the family. Daily hospital visits are reduced. We use technology to monitor vital parameters and the results are collated and conveyed to the attending doctor on a daily basis, if needed.'

Many such ventures have sprouted across the country, ensuring better homecare and reduced hospitalization.

Most of these activities come under the umbrella of health education and not necessarily medication, a point I explore further in the next chapter. Do we really need more hospitals for these activities?

Risks of hospitalization

Hospitalization is not without inherent risks. Hospital-related infections are a real threat to patients across the globe. If a patient is admitted into a hospital for a cardiac problem and then contracts a UTI, it can be attributed to an infection acquired during or post-hospitalization.

> HAIs are quite common in India but we still do not have national data for the number of infections across the country. A WHO report on HAI states:[8]

- Out of every 100 patients, 7 in high- and 15 in low-/middle-income countries (LMIC) will acquire at least one HAI, in acute care hospitals.
- 1 in every 10 affected patients dies of HAI.
- 8.9 million HAIs occur every year in acute and long-term care facilities in the European Union / European Economic Area.

Some examples of these infections include:

- Methicillin-Resistant Staphylococcus Aureus (MRSA): germs can enter the patient's bloodstream through a catheter or a medical tube inserted in the patient's vein, leading to an infection in the blood.
- Catheter Associated Urinary Tract Infections (CAUTI): infections caused by a urinary catheter.
- Surgical Site Infections (SSI): simple skin infections around the surgical site or deeper infections in the tissues or organs around the surgical area.
- Ventilator-Associated Pneumonia (VAP): pneumonia caused by germs entering the lungs through the ventilator tubes.
- Clostridium Difficile Infections (CDIs): Diarrhoea that lasts for a long time because of overuse of antibiotics, especially in the senior population.

Sepsis, an overwhelming infection leading to failure of organ systems, is a common side-effect of long-term hospitalization and is one of the leading causes of death in hospitals.

These infections are often caused by poor hygiene, not following protocols and undertrained and overworked hospital workers.

The risks are not limited to physical health. It also leads to significant emotional issues. Irrespective of the kind of hospital, a stay there induces emotional stress in patients and their caregivers, not to mention the financial stress. Hospitalization has been known to exacerbate feelings of depression and anxiety amongst patients. The story of Anirudh Manuskhani* is heartbreaking. His mother, Kshama Manuskhani,* recounts, 'Anirudh was admitted for removing his tonsils. He was to stay in the hospital overnight and since we could not afford a single room, we admitted him to a common ward. He was a lively ten-year-old, and it was difficult keeping him calm and in the bed. In the few hours he was there, he ran around, making friends with everyone—patient, caregiver, nurse—no one escaped his charms. We managed to drag him back to his bed and keep him there, threatening him with dire consequences if he ran around. Chastened, he settled in for some time and was dozing off when a child a few beds away went into some kind of emergency. The room was filled with nurses and doctors and as they were wheeling the child out of the room, the child passed away. There was a lot of chaos in the room as the family members started wailing and shouting. The hospital team tried to calm them down but the family only increased their outburst of grief. A couple of them accused the medical staff of negligence and it soon became a free-for-all. The other patients in the ward were petrified and some of the children started to cry. I couldn't take Anirudh out of the room as the entrance was blocked by an irate crowd. Anirudh was inconsolable and refused to be wheeled into the surgery room the next day. The doctor suggested that we sedate him for a bit and then attempt the procedure after a week or so.

'This was more than eleven years ago. Anirudh has still not recovered from that shock. He slipped into a deep depression and has even attempted self-harm a couple of times. I don't know what will happen to him once my time is up.'

Anirudh's case is extreme. But we cannot ignore the psychological and emotional experiences of hospitalization, an area that is often overlooked.

An ageing patient population and their needs

People are living longer than ever before. And people are also contracting health issues at much younger ages. It is no longer a surprise to see a family with a nonagenarian grandparent with age-related issues, a septuagenarian parent with a chronic ailment and a grandchild in their thirties with an autoimmune condition or chronic pain. In this scenario, who will be the caretaker?

A sizeable proportion of the elderly now opt for non-invasive treatment options towards the end of their lives, thus also reducing the load on hospitals. Dr Balraj Bhatt,* who works in critical care, says, 'In the last few years, I have noticed a big surge in the number of patients signing DNR [do not resuscitate] forms on admission to the ICU. Elderly patients refusing ventilators or invasive therapy in ICUs is now almost the norm. This means that ICU stays tend to be less prolonged in cases of poor outcomes. I feel that, today, people are willing to let go rather than hang on to life—a life that is most likely of poor quality with the ravages of age and disease—by a thread and die a slow death after incurring substantial costs.'

This is an incredibly significant point. This change in mindset means that ICUs may not be overburdened with cases of poor outcomes. Another significant aspect is the emergence of palliative care centres and hospices, which shifts end-of-life care from hospitals to these centres or even to patients' homes.

A changing workforce

Doctors, nurses, midwives, Accredited Social Health Activist (ASHA) workers, technicians are all part of the healthcare workforce. There are 13,01,319 allopathic doctors registered with state medical councils and the NMC, as of November 2021. The doctor–population ratio is 1:834 in the country, assuming 80 per cent availability of registered allopathic doctors and 5.65 lakh Ayurveda, yoga and naturopathy, unani, siddha and homeopathy, or AYUSH, doctors. Also, there are 2.89 lakh registered dentists, 32.63 lakh registered nursing personnel and 13 lakh allied healthcare professionals in the country.[9] These numbers seem significant on their own but, considering our population, we need many more skilled people to join the workforce. Hospitals in India are struggling to attract and retain talent across all levels.

Even before the pandemic, it was not an easy life for a healthcare worker. Insane working hours, not enough money, no work–life balance, high levels of stress and mental health issues are part of the workday of an average healthcare worker, regardless of the line of work.

Rural and remote areas struggle to find qualified professionals. The response to this challenge has been building more teaching institutions. But is that a solution?

The Karnataka government started around eight institutes in the middle of the last decade with the aim to ensure that every district has a tertiary medical care unit. Noble intentions, indeed. A few facts about this venture:[10]

- Karwar Institute of Medical Sciences was started in 2017 and still does not have cardiology and neurology departments.
- Koppal Institute of Medical Sciences, established in 2019, is still looking for land to construct a building.
- Haveri Institute of Medical Sciences functions out of an engineering college's building.

It is not just colleges in the interiors that are facing shortages. As of March 2023, 363 doctors and faculty member posts and 1,055 paramedic posts are lying vacant at the All-India Institute of Medical Sciences (AIIMS), New Delhi.[11]

Aravind Eye Hospitals has expanded the use of technicians in the operating room to assist surgeons with specific tasks, which enables the latter to be more efficient and treat many more patients. Today, technicians make up about 60 per cent of their workforce. In addition, Aravind has expanded the role of its nurses, which it calls mid-level ophthalmic personnel, to perform all hospital tasks other than operations and diagnoses.[12]

Technology does come to the rescue at times but it cannot be the answer to all the problems. What is the logic in building institutions when there is no one to teach or even work there?

Why, Then, Do We Build More Hospitals and Medical Institutes?

In India, we still speak of hospital bed to population ratios and doctor to population ratios without taking into account changing trends in healthcare delivery. As mentioned earlier, the present hospital bed to population ratio in India is 1 bed for every 1,000 people and the aim is to get it to 3 beds for 1,000 people. Obviously, we need more hospitals. But we do not need more in urban areas, where the hospitals of the future are going to see fewer footfalls as smart medicine and technology keeps more patients in their homes.

We need more hospitals in underserved areas. But how do we staff these hospitals? And what good is an understaffed hospital?

One of the reasons hospitals keep getting built in India though they may be understaffed, poorly equipped and may provide an awful level of care is due to the curse of visible spending in healthcare, as we have seen in the earlier chapters. Another reason is that there are sizable kickbacks to be made from issuing large building contracts. Everyone in the government loves promising big buildings. They can be shown to people as proof of 'development' in the area, and with money to be made on the side, it makes for an irresistible combination.

A hospital at the best of times is a dangerous place, and a poorly staffed, ill-equipped hospital can be a killing field. Without the right personnel and equipment, they can be a threat to life. Patients are simply unaware of this. Neither the government that builds them nor the people who seek treatment there realize that big buildings with vitrified tile flooring and snazzy interiors do not mean better healthcare.

Those who speak up for the need for more hospitals point to India's large corporate hospitals continuing to add bed capacity at a brisk rate. They are betting their money on hospitals staying as relevant as ever. They also point to the increasing percentage of the population that can afford better quality healthcare in India.

One trend that has undoubtedly been noticed is the shift of patients to the bigger hospital groups. This has led to the small hospitals and nursing homes, where the vast majority of hospital beds in India are, losing clients, especially in the large cities. Across India, hundreds of small hospitals and nursing homes are shutting down unable to face competition from the large hospitals and struggling to fill beds.

The COVID-19 pandemic saw a rapid increase in hospital bed capacity. However, this was largely in government hospitals. The private sector mostly redeployed their existing beds to deal with COVID-19 patients. Many of the beds added by the government remain vacant today and are unlikely to find occupants, barring another unforeseen pandemic.

The silver lining for hospitals is that India is expected to have a much higher proportion of senior citizens in the coming decades. With life spans increasing and lifestyle diseases taking over from infectious diseases as the major driver of disease burden, hospitals in India still see potential for further growth.

The spoiler could be healthcare technology, where disruptive advancements can put paid to the best laid plans of hospital heads. Will the hospital as we know it today even survive in the future, say, fifty years from now?

If Not Hospitals, Then What?

Technology will continue to disrupt this sector and bring about even more radical changes in the way patient care is administered. Robotics, artificial intelligence (AI), precision medicine, telemedicine, wearable devices, data collection and sharing—these areas will continue to grow.

The homecare industry will also expand, and community care will be the future. For patients, this means lower expenses, as well as better convenience and comfort. Hospitals will save on physical infrastructure and thus will be able to utilize their resources more effectively, reducing costs significantly.

The focus will necessarily turn to education rather than treatment, forcing largescale public health reforms.

As for doctors and surgeons, they will need to be experts at using technology. AI-powered tools will become the doctor's best friend. AI can analyse reams of data and detect patterns and anomalies and suggest diagnosis options. Doctors can then interpret these and finalize the optimal treatment plan.

Of course, I am not even remotely suggesting that hospitals will cease to exist. They are an integral part of the healthcare delivery system, and a vital one at that. All I am saying is that the structures of hospitals as we know them now will change. According to a few experts, the hospitals of the future may be 80 per cent service and 20 per cent physical location.

My friend B.G. Menon, Managing Director of ACME Consulting, which specializes in healthcare quality and performance improvement, offers this solution: 'Indian companies have a huge CSR budget. We need to harness this into healthcare investment. Let a corporation adopt an area and build a hospital and other facilities like schools around it. The doctors and other staff in this hospital can be paid competitively. The corporation can assist in managing the hospital and making it self-sustainable. Since it is run as a CSR activity, the end goal is not profitability but service to the local population. This model can be easily replicated even in the remote areas of the country.'

Though this is a great model on paper, I am not sure about its feasibility as CSR budgets tend to fluctuate, and corporate priorities are prone to change with their business needs. While I am not sure of the viability and scalability of this model, it would be interesting to try it out in a few areas around the country before we rule it out.

The powers-that-be will be forced to rethink their healthcare philosophy and make some drastic changes in the way they operate in the future. The sooner they realize this, the better it is for you and me.

10

Public Health: The Unfortunate Orphan

Have you heard of the Indian town of Gorakhpur? This town in Uttar Pradesh has the dubious distinction of being the encephalitis capital of the world since 1978, when the first known cases were reported.[1] From that time, around 25,000 deaths have been recorded. The actual number may be anywhere upwards of 50,000.[2]

And the major reason for the spread of this disease? Poor sanitation and poor nutrition. Mosquitoes that breed in stagnant and dirty water spread the virus that causes encephalitis. Malnourished children are more susceptible to its effects. This epidemic would have gone unnoticed if it was not for the death of sixty-three children which occurred when the state-run Baba Raghav Das Medical College hospital ran out of piped oxygen. This created a national and international furore and brought the town under the spotlight. As is their wont, the powers-to-be went on a damage control spree and started implementing some public health measures to prevent further outbreaks. But isn't it too little too late for the families who lost their children to this deadly yet preventable disease?

These deaths could not have been prevented by doctors. The only way these could have been prevented was through stringent public health policies.

Public health encompasses efforts made to improve the health of a broad population with investments not ordinarily considered 'healthcare'—for example, ad campaigns that encourage healthy behaviours, like exercising or quit smoking; or efforts to improve housing and nutrition for low-income populations or the quality of air or drinking water for everyone. Public health reduces the need to see a doctor by ensuring that the individual stays healthy.

A few successful public health gains include vaccination, planned parenthood, increased workplace safety measures and so on.

Logic says that every government should be focusing on public health. Increased public health services obviously will mean less sickness. But the reality is that no one wants to be in public health. Why are governments reluctant to increase public health spending? Is public health relegated to the background to help the healthcare industry thrive? After all, the industry profits only if there is sickness!

Public Health Authorities Caught Napping

Menstruation is one of the most taboo subjects across India. A normal biological process is considered unholy and dirty. Women are often shunned during their monthly cycles. With changing food habits and other reasons, girls are attaining puberty at an earlier age and would need safe and hygienic products to use during their cycles. However, not many can afford expensive sanitary napkins. Cloth is often used instead. But without access to water, it is extremely difficult to clean the cloth napkins properly. Many women living in abject poverty cannot afford to have individual pieces of cloth and end up sharing the same piece among them. This leads to vaginal infections that may affect their fertility.

The past couple of years has seen an upsurge in home delivery platforms. Companies like Swiggy, Zomato and others have exploded in popularity, with each one vying to offer cheaper and better service to the consumer. Take a moment to think about these delivery people. They work continuously and without a break. Most of them are in their mid-twenties and you can often see them around the local paan shop buying a cigarette or chewing tobacco. When I asked one of them as to why they chew so much tobacco, he said, 'Sir, I don't get time to eat. When I chew tobacco, my hunger gets killed and I can work longer and earn more.'

In a country where top film stars endorse the use of a product which is known to cause cancer, what can you say to these poor youths? While the product in question is glamourized as 'elaichi', everyone knows that the actual product is ghutka.

I read a recent report about the health of children of construction workers: they are malnourished but overweight. How does this happen? These workers often travel across the country and work in unsafe environments. The children are left to their own devices. Both men and women work in this industry, and they often do not have a kitchen. They survive on food from nearby vendors—buns, chips, sugary foods and the occasional banana constitutes their daily diet. While this diet satiates their hunger, it provides limited nutrition, leading to obesity and many other diseases like early-onset diabetes.

These are just a few examples of the consequences of public health authorities turning a blind eye to an obvious and massive problem. Everyone falls victim to this lackadaisical approach. How can a country expect to succeed if a large percentage of its population is unhealthy?

How Did Public Health Evolve in the Western World?

The WHO defines public health as 'the art and science of preventing disease, prolonging life and promoting health through the organized efforts of society'.[3]

Any activity conducted by governments to reduce exposure to disease for the general population falls under the purview of public health. Governments must ensure that their population has access to clean drinking water and safe food. Managing strict hygiene protocols and educating the population on improving and maintaining personal health also fall under this umbrella. Public health activities include vaccination and inoculation—but experts opine that non-medical activities do much more in ensuring a healthy populace than medical interventions.

The modern public health system is highly influenced by advances in medicine. As scientists studied the reasons behind many disease outbreaks, they found a strong link between hygiene and the prevalence of disease. Even two centuries ago, there was a largely fatalistic attitude towards disease and the focus was more on curing a disease-afflicted person. There is some anecdotal evidence of how rulers of individual kingdoms in India would resort to large-scale prayers and yagnas to control outbreaks of diseases.

By the late seventeenth century, European cities appointed public authorities to enforce isolation and quarantine protocols to avoid widespread outbreaks of contagious diseases.[4] The eighteenth century witnessed measures by governments to strengthen these practices, and official committees were formed to develop public health guidelines. Environmental pollution reared its ugly head in the early nineteenth century, with rapid industrialization in Europe and America. Lakes and rivers became polluted, and mountains of garbage and filth started to pile up in cities. Isolation and quarantine measures were not enough at this juncture as diseases like smallpox, typhoid, cholera and tuberculosis invaded the population. The earlier hypothesis that these diseases emerged from other shores and were brought into the country by travellers was challenged, and it became clear that the source of the outbreak emanated from within. As governments struggled to cope with never-ending epidemics, it became clear that measures needed to be taken to prevent outbreaks rather than control them after the fact.

Though immunization programmes and sanitization methods were adopted by the early twentieth century in the US, they weren't enough. A large part of the poorer population was still affected by these conditions, either because of lack of facilities or ignorance. Public health officials started to focus on health education for individuals and ran various health campaigns to educate the public at large. The role of public health was defined as 'the science of preventing contagious disease, prolonging life, and promoting physical health and efficiency'.[5]

The Nordic countries (Denmark, Norway, Sweden, Finland, and Iceland; the autonomous territories of Faroe Islands and Greenland; and the autonomous region of Aland) feature consistently in the list of countries with the best public health policies. This is not just because of their relatively smaller sizes and lower populations; Nordic welfare is built on the idea of good health for all. The basic values underpinning the model are compassion, tolerance and the conviction that all humans are of equal worth.[6]

Nordic principles of openness, transparency and freedom of expression are widely acclaimed. Because of this, their citizens trust their fellow citizens and official agencies and are willing to pay more tax to fund welfare provisions.

These countries operate on the principle that while citizens have the right to receive help from the government, they are also expected to contribute to the society. The ability to continually adapt to new challenges is a prerequisite for preserving the Nordic model and for coming up with innovative new welfare solutions. Universal initiatives have enabled these countries to combat infectious diseases through vaccinations and to make significant progress in combating lifestyle diseases via alcohol policies and smoking bans.

How Did the Movement Start in India?

British officials in India took a leaf out of their counterparts' book in Britain and implemented public health policies in colonial India. These activities were often limited to protecting British citizens and those working for the British. Colonial privilege meant that the chosen few lived in segregated and well-sanitized areas, while the larger population was ignored. In their quest to protect themselves, the British built capacity for delivering public health services (like the Calcutta School of Tropical Medicine), introduced legislations similar to those in their home country, founded sanitary departments for civilians answerable directly to the government, and focused on research for policymaking and planning for public health services. Even with these limited measures, there was a significant decrease in mortality rates from epidemics like cholera and the plague. But diseases like malaria and gastroenteric infections continued to haunt the population.

Post-Independence India had many challenges, and public health soon slipped further and further back in the list of priorities. In the 1950s, public health services were merged with medical services. Top posts in public health were filled by people with no background in the field and curative skills were rewarded over public health skills. This started the slow decay of the Indian public health system.

It is also interesting to note that the Indian Constitution does not specifically mention the right to healthcare as a fundamental right. Article 47 of the Constitution of India states:[7]

> Duty of the State to raise the level of nutrition and the standard of living and to improve public health: The State shall regard the raising of the level of nutrition and the standard of living of its people and the improvement of public health as among its primary duties and, in particular, the State shall endeavour to bring about prohibition of the consumption except for medicinal purposes of intoxicating drinks and of drugs which are injurious to health.

Unfortunately, this is considered more of a directive than a binding order by the central and state governments.

According to the Global Health Observatory, the data repository of the WHO, the 2018 current health expenditure (CHE) as percentage of GDP for India was 3.54 per cent, which is lower than Nepal (5.84 per cent) and Sri Lanka (3.76 per cent).[8]

I believe that one of the reasons for the devastating second wave of the COVID-19 pandemic in India was because the government treats public health as an unwanted, unloved orphan.

The leaders of the newly founded Republic of India had many challenges. Centuries of colonial rule had left the economy crippled. There was a wide gap in the education levels of people. The British rulers' approach to public health meant that the larger Indian population was left to fend for itself. The first Five-Year Plan (1951–56) found that only 3 per cent of Indian households had toilets, and the majority of the population lacked basic services like clean water, drainage and waste disposal systems. The focus of consecutive Five-Year Plans was on economic and industrial development, and less on filling the above gaps for citizens. While India has truly emerged as a force to be reckoned with, it is reprehensible that even as late as 2015, almost 5.2 crore people were defecating in the open.[9] I have collated some of the reasons for why we are in this situation.

As India invested in improving medical facilities, the focus was on building hospitals and increasing the reach of primary medical care across the country. While building hospitals is a noble cause, it does not address the basic issue of prevention. Various policymakers have unfortunately confused primary healthcare with public health activities. Primary healthcare can help a patient if they are diagnosed with malaria. Public health activities can ensure that the outbreak of malaria in the area is contained or even prevented by ensuring proper water drainage systems.

Popular wins over strategic measures

India is a democratic country. This means that the leaders of various governing agencies are elected by voters, who are swayed by promises of a better future. Who would you vote for? Someone who promises to build a hospital in your village or someone who promises to run awareness campaigns to prevent the rapid spread of non-communicable diseases, like diabetes?

The curse of visible spending in healthcare ensures that buildings and medical equipment get a disproportionately larger budget allocation in healthcare. This myopic way of working lends itself to confusion and competition among various departments. For example, the central government may focus on building toilets. The funds allocated to the various states are linked to this project and local governments have little freedom to reallocate them to more burning issues in their area.

Woefully dated laws and governing structures

As mentioned earlier, the Indian constitution does not clearly include healthcare as a fundamental right and has largely left the task of running public health campaigns to the discretion of the states. It is also interesting to note that many of the public health acts have not been updated since the British era.

Nexus between industry and politics

The nexus between the healthcare industry and the various people in power has played a major role in further overlooking public health activities. For example, diarrhoea is still a major cause of death in India. One of the treatments for diarrhoea is oral rehydration solution (ORS). This can easily be made in every home. But the healthcare industry has taken over this concept and mints a sizable amount of money selling preformulated ORS packages. Even today, there is a great deal of ignorance about diarrhoea, with many still believing that children with the condition should not be fed at all.

If there are enough funds allocated for strong public health campaigns, I believe that we can prevent the lakhs of deaths due to diarrhoea.

Paucity of competent human resources

Urmi is an ASHA worker in the state of Maharashtra. ASHA workers were deployed by the government from 2005 under the National Rural Health Mission (NHRM). The mission document defines these workers as 'honorary volunteers' who will be paid a performance-linked salary for their contribution in promoting immunization campaigns, sanitation measures and any other healthcare delivery programmes. Urmi was thrilled when she was recruited for this job and was told that she would be paid a monthly amount of ₹8,500. Little did she realize that the quantum of work and expectations from the higher-ups would squeeze her will to live. She says, 'I have two children of my own and live with an ailing father-in-law and a stubborn mother-in-law. My husband is a farmer. We haven't seen a good crop for years now. I thought that this income would help me feed my children. I wake up every day at around 4 a.m. and rush to finish all the household chores before I go out into nearby villages. I travel by bus to each village. As there are only a few buses in the area, I often need to wait an hour for one. I wish I had a bicycle, but where is the money to buy one? I go from house to house explaining the need for vaccines, building toilets, etc. While some people treat me with respect, many laugh at me. The village lads tease and taunt me or come and talk to me about unspeakable things. I have to grit my teeth and bear it all for the salary. I have to work in all weather conditions. While no one appreciates my presence, if I miss work for even one day, I am penalized. During the worst of the pandemic, I was supposed to still go from house to house. I was given a single mask and a pair of gloves. I contracted the virus and my family members refused to allow me into the house. I slept in a shed. And there is no appreciation from the authorities. After all this, my salary was not paid for nearly five months. But I couldn't quit as I needed the money and was hoping that I would get paid someday. One day, my husband beat me up accusing me of having an affair—why would I go to work despite no pay? I am told that someone called the WHO recognized our services and gave all of us an award. I wish they would give us money instead!'

There is a dearth of public health professionals in India across all levels. As mentioned earlier, after Independence, the reins of public health governance were handed over to medical professionals who worked under the premise that medicine had all the answers. This meant that the approach to any campaign was focused on arriving at a treatment than on educating the population.

Public health employees at the grassroots do not have it easy. For example, many positions of sanitary inspectors are vacant because their salaries have to come in from state government funds, and states are often financially strapped. The central government supports the family planning programme and hence funds the salaries of many female health workers. There are instances of people in senior positions who have received little or no training in public health. Is it any wonder, then, that most decisions are taken in a non-scientific and ad hoc manner? Public health is also seen as a lower form of medicine and so doctors are reluctant to sign up for it as a specialty.

Let us look at some numbers.[10] Between 1997 and 2017, the number of institutions offering Master of Public Health programmes increased from two to forty-four. But in 2016–17, only 704 students were enrolled out of the 1,190 available seats, a place occupancy of 59 per cent. How do we expect to meet the needs of the population with such a low enrolment rate? The irony is that this gap exists not because we do not have the resources, but because the resources do not find public health jobs appealing!

Working at cross-purposes

Many government departments have fine-tuned the art of zero inter-departmental communications. For example, the irrigation department of a zilla may embark on a canal project. Many times, such projects are left unfinished for reasons that are known only to the department. This becomes a breeding ground for mosquitoes and the health department in the area might be blissfully unaware of the situation until the local hospital reports the outbreak.

Losing steam when 75 per cent of goals are achieved

I sometimes feel that, as a country, we are quick to pat ourselves on our backs as soon as we see a little success. While this may serve as a motivator, this attitude also leads to complacency. Campaigns are started all the time, but as soon as we witness some success, the focus shifts to other areas. The second wave of COVID-19 is a prime example. All COVID-19 protocols like wearing masks, ensuring social distancing and frequent handwashing and sanitization were largely ignored as the numbers of the first wave declined. With the focus shifting to vaccination, we were lulled into a false sense of security.

Government priorities change with regimes as politicians want the publicity and accolades that come in with launching new schemes or programmes. Many such initiatives that were started by earlier governments have been halted midway to give way to new ones.

Missing the forest for the trees

One of our most enduring public health campaigns has been in the area of population control. Many of my generation would recall the forced sterilization activities that were conducted during the infamous Emergency of 1975. It did raise a lot of hackles, but it brought the issue of population control to the forefront. Since then, subsequent governments have introduced many schemes to curb the rapid increase of population. But with all the best will in the world, we still have some distance to go when it comes to controlling our population. While the two-child norm is more or less accepted in urban, educated India, this is still not the case in many parts of the country. Lakhs continue to procreate even after conceiving multiple children because, in their view, the higher the number of children (preferably sons), the higher the chances of prosperity. Population control is linked to other factors like education—especially of girls—employment, sanitary living conditions, etc. This is an issue of ideology and beliefs and that is what a smart campaign should address. Campaigns focusing on female literacy may have achieved more in the area of population control than the family planning programmes themselves. One of the reasons may be that a large section of the population still believes that more children mean more prosperity. Many men are reluctant to undergo sterilization as they believe that it would reduce their physical strength. Other forms of sterilization are not widely accepted. Educating women also means that they can make more informed decisions regarding the size of the family and use appropriate birth control methods.

When Public Health Succeeded

The response to the 1994 plague in Surat is a great example of how public health officials stepped in and turned the entire situation around.[11] Back in 1994, Surat had a population of approximately 14 lakhs, with 40 per cent being migrants, of which 80 per cent lived in slums. The city was known for its textiles and diamond cutting units and flourished economically. However, the infrastructure of the city was not geared to meet the needs of this huge population. There were no proper garbage collection methods, drainage systems or clean drinking water available to much of the population. Even before 1994, the city had frequent epidemics of malaria, gastroenteritis, cholera, dengue and hepatitis. It doesn't take a rocket scientist to make the connection between unhygienic conditions and these frequent outbreaks. Heavy rainfall led to flooding, and as the floods receded, the roads were piled up with bodies of dead rats and garbage. The local government was not prepared for this and hadn't organized proper cleanup. This was a starting point for the plague.

Panic and chaos ensued, not only in the city but also in other states, such as Maharashtra and Andhra Pradesh, due to the rapid spread of misinformation. The lack of coordination between various government bodies lead to health officials declaring it as an epidemic of plague without knowing whether it was pneumonic.

Within two years of this outbreak, Surat was recognized as one of the cleanest cities in India. How did this transformation happen? All it needed was an official who used public health as a basis for all his activities. Municipal Commissioner S.R. Rao led his team to work on improving sanitization, building toilets, creating special garbage disposal areas and bringing down illegal construction. He managed to bring this change without any significant additional state or central government aid. His team educated the residents on proper hygiene and urged citizens to dispose of household waste properly. The transformation in Surat exemplifies the fact that public health is everybody's business, not just the health department's. For the department to succeed, it needs to work with all the other local governments, engineering, water supply, civil works, sanitation, etc. If you need further proof that public health can make a difference, you need not look further than the drop in the cases of malaria in Surat, from 21,540 in 1994 to 7,734 in 2014.[12] Surat today consistently features in the top ten list of cleanest cities in India in the Swachh Survekshan survey.

Another example of public health success is the Pulse Polio Programme. It is a stellar example of what can be achieved with political will and when governments, civic bodies, NGOs and other organizations work in tandem.

In March 2014, the WHO declared India as a polio free country, an achievement that needs to be applauded. It is estimated that, before 1980, around 2 lakh children were crippled each year by the polio virus.[13] Eradication of polio became the focal point of public health, with India becoming a signatory to the Global Polio Eradication resolution passed in 1988.

The year 1994 witnessed a mass immunization campaign in New Delhi, covering almost 10 lakh children under the age of three. Following its success, national immunization days (NIDs) were conducted twice a year across the country, and multiple rounds of sub-national immunization days (SNID) were conducted in high-risk areas.

To ensure that children benefited from the Oral Polio Vaccine, community mobilizers educated parents on the need for hygiene and sanitation to prevent bouts of diarrhoea. Vaccination booths were set up across India. Employees and volunteers were trained on the administration of the vaccine. Apart from fixed vaccination centres, bus stops, railway stations, international borders with high volumes of immigrants, airports and schools were also covered. Door-to-door campaigns were held in villages and remote areas. Parents and guardians were urged to bring in their children on NIDs and SNIDs even if the children were vaccinated. Systematic records were maintained, and missing children were identified and vaccinated. Over the years, better vaccines were developed and administered to protect children from all strains of polio.

The last reported polio case in India was in 2011 of a two-year-old girl in Howrah, West Bengal.[14] The girl was often sick with diarrhoea, and her parents were not prepared to vaccinate her despite the best efforts of the community workers. Within seven days of the case being reported, the Indian government launched a large-scale mop-up immunization campaign. The aggressive response succeeded, and India is now proudly polio free!

Public Health beyond Communicable Diseases

While we have made considerable progress in the management of communicable diseases, non-communicable diseases (NCD) have emerged as the leading causes of death globally. These can include chronic respiratory conditions because of poor air quality, liver conditions due to alcohol, cancer due to tobacco usage and heart conditions and diabetes linked to unhealthy food and lifestyle. Mental health is also another neglected issue that increasingly needs greater attention among almost all age groups and strata of society.

The 2019 country report[15] on India by the Institute for Health Metrics and Evaluation (IHME) reveals that in just ten years, NCDs have replaced communicable diseases as the top causes of death. In 2009, the three top killers were ischemic heart disease, diarrhoeal diseases and neonatal diseases. In 2019, the three top killers were ischemic heart disease, chronic obstructive pulmonary disease and strokes.

This increase in NCDs has a larger impact on society. Chronic conditions lead to reduced quality of life and are an additional burden on society. These diseases are no longer the sole burden of the affluent—they affect the poorest of the poor.

Why is India considered to be the golden goose for the healthcare industry? All these new patients with NCDs will need prolonged care and hence contribute to the bottom line of the industry. According to me, this is the time to step up public health activities. Raising awareness is just one part of the solution. The main part is to understand the social context of these diseases and address those issues. The link between unclean food, air and water with diseases is well-proven. But how many towns have all of this? Every year, come winter, there is a furious debate about the abysmal quality of air in the national capital. But where are the concrete steps taken to control this situation? What about the rampant use of pesticides in food production? While there are rules in place, where are the systems to ensure adherence? A firm political will beyond just vote-catching tactics is required to stem the rot and put public health before sheer greed.

Where Does One Go from Here?

Vaccination process too slow? Urban planning all over the place? Lack of clean water for all? The answer to all our problems, according to many pundits, lies in privatization. Take the onus away from the governments and give it to the private industries. After all, there are many shining examples of how privatization has given us a higher standard of living. Tempting as it may be, I think we need to take a step back and look at the issue from all angles before taking this step.

There has been a lot of study on the impact of privatization of public health services. And many researchers have concluded that across the world, reforms under the guise of ensuring efficiency, quality, services improvement, etc., have actually boomeranged and further debilitated public healthcare systems. This has led to further commercialization of care. In this Catch-22 situation, the case is reinforced for privatization of public healthcare systems.

Entities like the World Bank, the IMF and others contest that privatization will help governments reduce public expenditure and provide better health systems to all citizens. But what about factors like equity, equality and accessibility of healthcare for the poorest of the poor?

The city of Detroit in the US witnessed a major economic downturn from the 1990s through the 2000s. As the city geared towards filing for bankruptcy, its local authorities decided to privatize and outsource public health services.[16] While other cities in similar situations privatized some of the work, Detroit outsourced essentially all the city's health services. Because of this, the residents were left with no political influence to protect them from basic threats. Those in power remained largely silent when the Water and Sewerage Department began shutting off services to households for non-payment or delayed payments. This affected the poorer communities who were already suffering from myriad issues. Experts opine, and I agree, that this would not have happened if it was not for the privatization of a public health department.

The COVID-19 pandemic has highlighted the many lacunae within our public health system. Citizens have been vociferous in their demand for change. Our current public health system needs sweeping reforms consistent with the new health realities. We need people with vision and will to change the system across all levels.

The hard truth is that public health is not sexy. It is gritty and demands tough action. The adage 'no man is an island' is proved painfully accurate in the field of health. One infected individual could easily start an epidemic if the disease is unchecked. Public boards, agencies, institutions and committees must be realigned and restructured with a single mission: to protect the health of the public.

Practices of good governance, productive partnerships between various agencies, accountability to the public and adoption of a preventative rather than curative approach can reenergize the public health system. Will the powers that be take heed and put public health on an even footing with the favored sibling—curative healthcare?

Annexure

Current Health Expenditure (CHE) as Percentage of GDP[17]			
Country	CHE	Country	CHE
Bangladesh	2.5	India	3
Pakistan	3.4	Sri Lanka	4.1
China	5.3	Russia	5.7
Brazil	9.6	UK	10.2
Japan	10.7	USA	16.8

Waste disposal in India[18]	Rural	Urban
per cent of people not using any type of toilet	33 per cent	4 per cent
per cent of people not disposing garbage properly (common place/ manure pit/ recycling)	54 per cent	10 per cent

11
Health Insurance in India

A few years ago, I suddenly felt a sharp pain in my abdomen. I was immediately rushed to a well-known corporate hospital. The attending doctor confirmed what I had feared: my appendix was severely inflamed and needed to be removed. The staff completed the initial formalities and scheduled the surgery. I was wheeled into the operating theatre. I emerged after a successful procedure and was then wheeled into the recovery room. At the time of discharge, I was presented with the bill; the total amount was about ₹1,10,000. I wasn't too worried—I had a good insurance policy from a reputed company.

When I submitted my claim, imagine my dismay when the insurance company informed me that they would only pay out ₹35,000! I was livid! I called up my insurance agent through whom I had purchased the policy. He listened patiently to the whole story and then said, 'Sir, I recommend that you don't accept their settlement. Let us file a complaint with the insurance ombudsman.' I agreed.

The ombudsman's office received my complaint and set a date for a hearing. My insurance agent, I and a representative of the insurance company were in attendance. The ombudsman listened to our case for all of five minutes, turned to the company representative and asked, 'What is your company's rate for an appendectomy at the hospital?' The rep excused himself to check with his superiors. A hurried phone call later, he returned to the room and said, 'At this hospital, for appendectomies, we cover up to ₹76,000.' The ombudsman shook his head and wrote out an order directing the insurance company to cover ₹76,000 of my hospital bill. Within two days, the company complied.

Between the surgery and the hearing, six whole months had passed.

I was shocked: a government-owned insurance company had tried to get away with paying less than half of what they were supposed to. And the only reason they were held to account was that I had refused to accept the initial settlement. If they could try this with me, how many others might have faced similar situations and given in because they didn't know how the system worked?

The Indian health system consists of a vast public health infrastructure and a generally unregulated private healthcare sector. Every year, lakhs of Indians are pushed into poverty because of out-of-pocket medical expenditures. Medical insurance helps but it is yet to penetrate across all socio-economic classes. Both government and private insurance providers have fallen short of providing real respite to most Indians. What is the real state of insurance in the country? How can the process be improved?

In this chapter, I discuss the health insurance system in India—how it functions, its effects on healthcare and the challenges faced by all parties involved.

Health insurance has come a long way in India in recent years. Many argue that it has been a critical tool for financing healthcare in the country, enabling access to quality medical care for lakhs of people who would otherwise have been unable to afford it. However, my own experience has shown the challenges that patients often face when navigating a system that was complicated even before adding the layers of network hospitals, copays, premium limits and out-of-pocket expenses to it.

What Is Health Insurance?

In the simplest terms, health insurance is a way of minimizing risk for the insured—the risk of having to pay huge medical bills in case of an unforeseen medical situation. The customer pays a fixed amount to the insurer, who, in return, promises to pay the customer's medical bills for a given period of time. The customer now gains peace of mind knowing that they won't have to foot massive medical bills.

If the customer doesn't face a medical emergency in the defined time period, the insurance company makes a profit. If the customer faces an emergency, the insurance company will face a payout that can be much more than what the customer has paid in premiums. So how does the insurance company mitigate the risk it is taking? Very simply, by selling insurance policies to large numbers of people.

> Here's an example:
>
> Company A offers a single policy: they will cover medical expenses of up to ₹1 lakh. Suppose the premium the customer pays for this policy is ₹1,000. If the company sells this policy to 10 lakh people, the company's income is:
>
> ₹1,000 x 10 lakh = ₹100 crores
>
> The company also knows that, of the customers buying the policy, only 5,000 of them are likely to face a medical emergency that they will need to cover. Thus, their expected payout is likely to be:
>
> ₹5,000 x 1 lakh = ₹ 50 crores
>
> This would net them a profit:
>
> ₹100 crores – ₹50 crores = ₹50 crores!
>
> Of course, this is a grossly oversimplified example. But it helps clarify a central concept: for insurance companies to be profitable, they need to do two things:
>
> - Increase the number of people covered, thus increasing premium collections and resulting in more income.
>
> - Reduce the number of claims that customers are likely to make, thus bringing down expenses.
>
> These two motivations drive some of the biggest challenges facing the healthcare ecosystem today.

The History of Health Insurance in India

Health insurance, as a concept, was introduced in India in the early 1900s.[1] The first health insurance scheme in India was started by the British Raj in 1912 for their civil servants. It provided coverage for hospitalization, maternity and surgery. The scheme was later extended to cover railway employees in 1923 and postal and telegraph employees in 1930.

In the post-Independence era, the Government of India started several health insurance schemes to provide healthcare coverage to the poor and the marginalized. One of the first such schemes was the Employees' State Insurance (ESI) scheme, which was launched in 1952. The scheme provided health insurance to employees in factories and industrial establishments, covering hospitalization, maternity and disability benefits. The scheme was later extended to cover dependents of the insured.

In 1986, the Government of India launched the Central Government Health Scheme (CGHS) to provide healthcare coverage to its employees and pensioners.

The 1990s saw the emergence of private health insurance in India. Since then, several private companies have entered the market, offering a range of health insurance products and services to individuals and groups.

In 2018, the Government of India launched the ambitious Ayushman Bharat, Prime Minister's Jan Aarogya Yojana, also known as the National Health Protection Scheme (NHPS), that would cover roughly the bottom 50 per cent of the country's population in terms of income. Under this plan, people will receive primary care from their existing doctors and can access secondary and tertiary healthcare for free, as required. Apart from this, most Indian states such as Tamil Nadu, Kerala, Telangana, etc., have their own health insurance schemes targeted towards residents in their jurisdictions. Some of these have now been merged into the Ayushman Bharat scheme.

The Current State of Health Insurance in India

The Indian health insurance market has grown significantly over the years. As of 2021, there are over thirty health insurance companies in India, offering a range of products and services to individuals and groups. The health insurance market in India is dominated by four major public sector insurance companies: National Insurance Company Limited, New India Assurance Company Limited, Oriental Insurance Company Limited and United India Insurance Company Limited.

This sector in India is regulated by the Insurance Regulatory and Development Authority of India (IRDAI). The IRDAI is responsible for ensuring that health insurance companies comply with the regulations and guidelines set by the government of India. It also regulates the premiums charged by health insurance companies and ensures that they are affordable for individuals and groups.

The challenges facing the insurance industry still loom large, however. According to the National Sample Survey of 2019,[2] 85.9 per cent of Indians in rural areas were without any health insurance coverage, whereas 80.9 per cent of urban Indians were uninsured. The launch of the Ayushman Bharat scheme has helped expand coverage: 22 crore verified beneficiaries and 4.3 crore hospital admissions have been authorized under this scheme as of January 2023.[3] However, considering that the scheme targets expanding benefits to 70 crore people, it's safe to say that there is still a long way to go.

Challenges Faced by Patients

Patients who visit a hospital are unlikely to be at their best mentally. Even the most well-informed and educated patient would find it difficult to negotiate the experience while dealing with pain, stress and illness. Some of the main challenges the patients face have been outlined below.

Complicated systems

At the hospital, most patients would find that availing their health insurance is a far more laborious process than advertised when the insurance is sold to them. They are often faced with jargon that means nothing to them: pre-existing conditions, copay, deductible, out-of-pocket, out-of-network, to name a few. At lower insurance levels, most tests require approvals from the insurer that need to be requested by the hospital, leading to delays while they wait to hear back. Navigating this system only adds to an already stressful experience.

Praful Wadekar,* a sixty-two-year-old man who was diagnosed with type 2 diabetes seventeen years ago, had a particularly jarring encounter with insurance-related red tape: 'Two years back, I switched insurance companies as I was getting a discount on the premium. This was after a hard sell from the company. They assured me that I would retain all the benefits of my previous plan. Despite a lot of care, I needed an amputation of my toe on the left foot. I was eligible for cashless admission but there was a problem at the time and I paid up thinking I could claim the amount later. I was more focused on my health and so were my family members. After the procedure was over and I was recovering at home, I submitted the claims. The claims were rejected without any reason. I tried calling the person who had sold the policy to me but his number was not operational. I called the customer service multiple times but was kept on hold continuously. When I did manage to reach the insurance company, I was informed that my request would not be honoured because diabetes was an undeclared pre-existing condition! How was that possible? I had clearly declared it in my application form when the representative was selling me the insurance. I was assured that the coverage would be continuous. I had a copy of the contract showing this declaration clearly. When I told them this, they put me on hold, and ten minutes later, asked me to email the complaint to them. We went back and forth over mails and calls and after six months, they released the payment. I was following up with them every second day and it was quite an effort. I was lucky that I had enough money to pay for the surgery at the time. What would someone who couldn't come up with that much money at short notice do? Also, not everyone would be so tenacious. Most people may just give up after a few calls. I call this sheer robbery!' he concludes angrily.

The fine print

Often, insurance contracts in India can contain some very strange stipulations that, quite simply, don't make any sense. Patients are often blissfully unaware that certain exceptions exist until these cases happen to them.

Srivatsa Rao,* a resident of Bangalore, shares his story: 'I am a cautious person and believe in insurance. My entire family including my parents and in-laws are covered under medical insurance with a leading private company. When my eighty-year-old father needed cataract surgery, we were not worried about our finances. After all, he had a ₹ 10-lakh cover, and the procedure was around ₹32,000 for each eye. Confident that it would be covered, we went ahead with the procedure. The right eye was operated first and the left after ten days. The insurance company covered the cost for the first eye but refused to cover for the second procedure. As I did not want to argue about this at the hospital, I paid the amount and brought my father back home. I called the insurance provider after a few days and I was told that according to the policy we had opted for, only the cost for one eye would be covered in a year. I was shocked at this absurdity and pointed out that I had been paying a decent premium for the last fifteen years and we had never availed of it, and this was the first time my father was hospitalized. The executive heard me out patiently but again politely told me that it was clearly mentioned in the policy document in the fine print and that she couldn't do anything about it. I was free to complain to the ombudsman, but since the policy document included this clause, it was unlikely that I would get any money from the company. How can we put our faith in insurance policies after this kind of experience?'

Difficulties in getting insurance for senior citizens

Sanjana Koppikar,* a thirty-three-year-old content creator says, 'My parents are both in their mid-seventies. Having lived in Canada for several years, they decided to move back to India to live out their retirements closer to home and family. We had been told how access to medical care was much better in India now, compared to the long waiting times to see even a general practitioner in Canada. So, they packed their lives up and moved to Mumbai. Initially, things were great. They found a consultant they were comfortable with and were regularly going to see him. The cost of healthcare and medication were a fraction of what they were used to be in Canada. They were, however, not eligible for insurance from most providers. At this point, given the low cost of healthcare we had experienced so far, we felt that we were well-prepared to deal with any medical expenses. However, the problems became apparent when my mother had to undergo a knee replacement.

'We approached an orthopaedic surgeon at a well-known corporate hospital who had a good track record with such procedures. The cost was a little higher than in other hospitals but still quite reasonable, we felt. On the day, she was checked in to the hospital and underwent the needed tests. The surgery itself seemed to go off without a hitch. Two days after the surgery, the attending physician who came to inspect the knee told my dad that there was a possibility of infection, and that my mother would have to spend a couple more days at the hospital under observation. They kept her in a hospital room for a week, ran a series of tests and put her on a course of antibiotics. When they were finally ready to discharge her, the bill was quite a shock! The post-surgery hospital stay cost as much as the procedure itself. Add to this several additional 'charges' such as a premium room, the food, equipment, etc., and the sum was quite eye-watering. When asked why they did not inform us of these charges beforehand, we were told that insurance usually covers all these, and they didn't know we were uninsured. I felt like the hospital was taking advantage of a pair of septuagenarians, who maybe would accept whatever they were told at face value. It was lucky that we could send money home to cover these expenses. What would a family without our resources do if confronted with a similar situation?'

Insurance companies are always trying to mitigate the risk of having to pay for customers' medical expenses. Therefore, while insurance for young people, such as those in their twenties, is cheap and readily available, things start getting much more expensive with age and pre-existing conditions. On a certain level, this is understandable—insurance companies exist to make money, after all.

But from the perspective of a customer who is looking to avoid being bankrupted by untimely medical bills, this is a disaster. Those who need it the least, such as the twenty-somethings mentioned above, can access insurance easily while the old and the infirm find it very hard to find health coverage. Most insurance companies do not even offer insurance to people over the age of seventy-five. Anyone with pre-existing conditions will find that their premium is several times higher than average. No wonder that the private insurance market is running at a loss—they are all competing for the same available customer base and trying to exclude those for whom medical care is actually critical.

It is hoped that programmes such as Ayushman Bharat, or Pradhan Mantri Jan Arogya Yojana (PM-JAY), and the various state health insurance programmes will help ease this burden somewhat by insuring those who require it, without a need to be profitable. However, as stated earlier, the coverage of these programmes still need to grow much further in order to reach their goals. These schemes are also plagued with a host of other problems, preventing them from being optimally effective.

Challenges faced by doctors, healthcare providers and health insurers

The advent of insurance has also added a new layer of bureaucracy to the already complex workings of a hospital.

Doctors now need to document their diagnoses according to standards set by the insurers if their claims need to be processed. Hospitals are now required to operate an insurance department to handle claims and payments.

The availability of insurance also makes doctors more likely to over-test and overtreat. According to Dr Noel Cherian,* a GP based out of Thiruvananthapuram, 'I've seen cases where patients who come to me with knee or joint pain are actually demanding surgery. Usually, these people are in their fifties who have been assured that the quickest way to get rid of the pain is through a knee replacement. Joint replacement is usually a drastic step, which is only taken after all other options such as physiotherapy and medication have failed. But now, you see cases where patients and doctors both treat it as a first line of treatment as the insurance will cover it. If the doctor refuses to perform the surgery, a lot of patients will just find someone else who will.'

On the other hand, the low rate of coverage in India poses strong challenges to the insurance industry itself. As we have seen before, insurance companies need large numbers of customers to effectively spread out the risk that they take. Basically, the problem is that there aren't enough customers for these companies to effectively reduce said risk. This can be seen in the financial numbers published by these companies. They have been facing losses for several years. Star Health, one of the biggest players in the market today, posted a loss of ₹1,040 crores in December 2022.[4]

One of the experts we spoke to opined that only 4 per cent of the population have individual medical insurance, while 11 per cent have insurance cover provided by their employers. Most people think that they don't need medical insurance as they are healthy. It is only when they have a sudden health emergency that they realize the importance of having a policy. Pankaja Ramakrishnan,* a thirty-three-year-old chef, says, 'I started working at the age of twenty-three. My father insisted that I take a life insurance policy and a health insurance policy. In the arrogance of youth, I refused. I was young, healthy and insurance is for old people like my parents. All was okay till my twenty-seventh birthday. I was in a cab, going to a restaurant to meet my friend to celebrate my birthday. I was sitting in the back with no seat belt and chatting away on my phone. Suddenly, there was a loud noise and when I opened my eyes, I was in a hospital with multiple fractures and injuries. I was in the hospital for almost a month and the bill ran into lakhs. All my savings were wiped out and I borrowed money from family and friends to meet the expenses. I was away from work for almost a year and had to move back in with my parents. I really wish that I had listened to my father.'

Insurance companies find it difficult to sell individual policies to the young population. Most people seem to go in for policies only after they develop a medical condition, by which time the pre-existing conditions clause of the plan kicks in.

Dr S. Prakash, former managing director, Star Health Insurance says, 'The best way to solve this is to make insurance more accessible to people. What the government and the people need to understand is that health insurance only gets better when the customer base grows. India, with its huge population and economic development, is in a good position to grow the customer base. This will ensure that companies like ours do not turn down customers for pre-existing conditions. The more people that subscribe, the better the service becomes for everyone. It is only then that we will be able to offer improved products similar to the ones available in advanced economies. And from a customer's perspective, it would greatly reduce the risk of going from above-the-poverty-line to below it due to a single unexpected medical condition.'

While government schemes like Ayushman Bharat are started with noble intentions, a lot of insurance companies have faced issues when working with these schemes. One important thing to note is that the implementation of these schemes varies from state to state, so the company has to establish and evolve new processes for dealing with each state agency. There have also been challenges in terms of getting paid on time, excessive red tape, etc. Unfortunately, due to these factors, several insurance companies choose to forego participation in these schemes. How can the scheme then reach more individuals?

Another key reason for the lack of profits in the insurance sector is insurance fraud. We can only presume what the actual numbers are as this is a very hard statistic to calculate. According to Dr Prakash, most studies put the leakage due to fraudulent claims between 12–17 per cent of all claims. If true, this has a massive impact on insurance companies' bottom line. Ever since insurance started covering laparoscopic surgeries, there has been a huge uptick in the number of gall-bladder removals and similar minor procedures. There has also been a huge increase in the number of ICU admissions claims. This is further complicated by the fact that there is no standard definition of ICUs—some ICUs in certain hospitals are nothing more than a glorified ward.

Dr Prakash believes that the only way to fix the problem is to come up with solutions by involving all the stakeholders—the patients, the hospitals, insurance companies and the government. 'Talking about the problem, I believe, is the correct first step. Only when there is an awareness of the problem can people think about solutions. The good thing is that there is a lot of expertise already available in the country. The challenge is to channel their skills to solve the issues we are facing now.'

There is not enough data on disease patterns in the country, so insurance providers struggle with product and pricing innovation.

All the success that has been achieved in the healthcare sector will be of no use unless its knowledge and expertise can be made available to all the citizens in the country. The first step towards this is to promote awareness among people as to why insurance is necessary. If even 50 per cent of India's population signs up for it, the industry as a whole will be able to contribute to much better healthcare service than we are seeing today. At that level, companies should routinely be able to offer products more suited to the needs of the individual, such as outpatient care, dental coverage, mental health, etc.

So, What Is the Solution?

Healthcare access even in advanced countries is plagued by issues.

Take for instance the US, where, if you have a good health insurance cover, you have access to the finest quality of care. Without it, even trivial investigations like an X-ray could cost upwards of $500. Or the UK, where the National Health Service, once held up as the model everyone should aspire to is crumbling under the twin challenges of rising demand and shrinking budgets and investment. You can find yourself waiting weeks to just see a GP.

In a country as vast as India, with its massive diversity in terms of socio-economic factors, is it even possible to build a healthcare model that provides equitable access to all its citizens? This is a daunting proposition, considering how thinly spread the country is in terms of healthcare infrastructure. However, the status quo is unsustainable, and this will drag down the development and progress of the country as a whole. So, how do we address this challenge? I suggest a seven-point approach.

- Government and private insurance providers need to work in partnership to build a health service that will truly benefit all the people.
- To standardize the cost of insurance, ensure consistent levels of care in hospitals across the country. With this achieved, the state and local governments will then work with Ayushman Bharat to integrate it with private insurers.
- Insurers can work through Ayushman Bharat to reach customers that are out of reach, increasing the customer base in the process. With parallel investments in healthcare, including a larger number of PHCs and secondary healthcare centres in rural areas, even the poorest of people will have adequate access to healthcare which will not result in crushing medical debt.
- The government and the IRDAI should set out clear guidelines and regulations on how insurance claims are to be treated. These guidelines should also remove unreasonable restrictions being buried in the fine print: the goal should be an insurance policy that can be understood without a law degree. Only then will the public feel that insurance is something that sets their minds at ease the next time they visit a hospital.
- Public education programmes about how insurance works, how the public benefits and what

to do in case they feel that the insurance company has not honoured their end of the contract are a must.

- Incentivize prevention, not treatment. Insurance companies need to graduate from covering procedures in hospitals to incentivizing people to have a proactively healthy lifestyle. Post-pandemic, we are seeing a lot of changes in disease profiles, with younger people getting affected by preventable chronic diseases. Providing incentives to live healthier lifestyles is an important evolution of health insurance.

- An integrated approach comprising of all stakeholders, all of whom are aligned to a clear goal, is the best way to ensure a healthy population.

12

Can AI-Supported Expert Systems Change the Face of Healthcare Delivery?

As a doctor, I have seen many patients experiencing adverse events after surgery. A patient dying after a successful operation is heartbreaking for both their family and the medical staff. Several of these deaths can be prevented by monitoring the patient and taking immediate action to counteract any signs of deterioration. Currently, monitoring is mostly done manually and hence is prone to human error. The workload of the nurses in the ward are also overstretched, and they find the process of entering data from the monitors and other medical devices into the hospital systems time-consuming.

As someone who is a technocrat and a doctor, I have had frequent discussions with my friends and colleagues on a possible solution. Most of these solutions sounded like something out of a science fiction novel! But many of these are now becoming a reality.

A few hospitals in the UK installed artificial intelligence (AI)-enabled tools in their wards. These tools automatically monitored vital signs, calculated early warning scores that signal possible patient deterioration and helped the care team to identify early signs of adverse events. This helps in providing a quick response, saving lives. One of these hospitals managed to reduce serious adverse events in the general ward by 35 per cent and cardiac arrests by a whopping 86 per cent.[1] Imagine the number of lives that could be saved if these tools are enabled across all hospitals around the world!

Technology has always partnered with healthcare to bring about significant improvements across all areas of healthcare delivery. In recent years, there is a lot of work happening in the field of AI, and this promises to usher in some revolutionary changes in the way the healthcare industry functions.

What is AI? Will it help diagnose and suggest treatments on par with or even better than doctors? Can AI help reduce the human error factor? Will it be adopted widely across clinical practices? What are the challenges in its adoption?

Read on to find answers to these questions.

What Is Artificial Intelligence ?

Unless you are a complete recluse or have no access to the internet, AI will not be a new term for you. While AI has been around in some form or the other for several decades, it only really entered the public consciousness in the early 2020s. The release of OpenAI's ChatGPT, a large language model or LLM (programs that can understand and generate human-like language), has helped showcase how far AI has come, and how it can be applied to everyday life.

This is a great example of AI but this is not the only one. When Amazon, Netflix, YouTube, Google, etc., throw recommendations to you, that is AI in action. Face recognition, voice recognition, interpreting images, etc., are again, the result of AI.

With all the buzz around AI, there is still a lot of confusion around what it is, exactly. I would define AI as the ability of a machine to perform cognitive functions such as learning, processing, decision-making, solving problems, etc., the way humans perform them. It doesn't matter how it is done—that is for the developers to decide. As consumers, we can't deny that our lives have been made easier because of AI.

AI encompasses a wide range of technologies, including machine learning, natural language processing, robotics and computer vision. Machine learning, in particular, has become increasingly popular in recent years and involves training computer algorithms to learn from data, rather than being explicitly programmed.

AI has revolutionized numerous industries, and healthcare is no exception. It has the potential to improve healthcare delivery by increasing efficiency, reducing errors and enhancing patient outcomes. In India, where a large gap exists between demand and supply of medical expertise and professionals, AI can be harnessed to redress this imbalance and significantly improve healthcare delivery, particularly in underserved regions where resources are limited.

Doctors and nurses are often stretched workwise and are fatigued after a long day. Not all of them are well-trained and efficient. Patient data is also not available easily. Most doctors in India still use pen and paper and rely on patients to maintain their health files. All these factors lead to misdiagnosis, improper treatment options, etc.

This is where AI supported systems save the day. Systems do not forget or get tired and can be updated with the latest guidelines. They help enhance levels of patient safety and are a huge asset in diagnosis.

A radiologist spends hours interpreting dozens of scans and X-rays in a working day. This process is time consuming and is prone to human error. Enter AI based systems. A hospital in Bengaluru uses such a system, developed by Qure.ai, and has managed to reduce the workload of radiologists. The scans and images are first read by the AI system and is categorized as normal or abnormal. It also flags images that may need human interpretation. Radiologists need to focus only on the second and third categories, thus saving a lot of time and reducing the margin of error.

I feel that by the end of this decade, such systems will become the norm for image interpretation in healthcare.

Applications of AI in Medicine

Clinical decision support systems (CDSS)

CDSS are computer tools that aid doctors in arriving at informed clinical decisions. They are one of the first cases of the use of AI in medicine. This has gone hand-in-hand with the adoption of Electronic Health Record (EHR) systems by medical practitioners and institutions. EHR data provides detailed information about the patient, including clinical notes, test results and lab values, which an algorithm can extract, analyse and compare with a dataset to deliver an accurate diagnosis of the patient's condition.

With the evolution of machine learning, widespread adoption of enabling technologies such as cloud computing and the abundance and easy access to powerful computer processors, AI has advanced in leaps and bounds. With the tighter integration of Decision Support Systems and EHRs into the clinical workflow, we expect this technology to advance at an exponential rate.

As I have mentioned many times in this book, hypertension and diabetes are the major health challenges in India. These diseases are no longer limited to the urban areas or to the senior population.

A group of researchers developed a model of care called Integrated Tracking, Referral, Electronic Decision Support and Care Coordination (I-TREC) that is calibrated for implementation within the current health system across all facility types.[2] They piloted this programme in a block in Shaheed Bhagat Singh Nagar district of Punjab.

They undertook an academic–community partnership to incorporate the combination of a CDSS with 'task-shifting'—a process where tasks like gathering the patient health history, can be shifted from doctors to the nurse/non-physician healthcare provider—into the Government of India's Non-Communicable Diseases System under the Comprehensive Primary Health Care System, a platform that assists healthcare providers to record patient information for routine NCD care. Academic partners developed clinical algorithms, conceptualized a revised clinic workflow and provided training modules with iterative collaboration and consultation with government and technology partners to incorporate CDSS within the existing system.

If this pilot succeeds, it will have a significant impact on the early diagnosis of a number of cases of these NCDs. It will also offer more effective treatment protocols at a lower cost. Learnings from I-TREC will provide a roadmap to other public health experts to integrate and adapt their interventions at the national level.

The advantage of CDSS is that it can be used on a variety of platforms, including personal computers, smartphones, wearables, electronic medical record networks, written material, etc. They can take many forms, from patient data summaries and computerized alerts, diagnostic and therapeutic protocols.

The purpose of CDSS is to improve the quality and safety of patient care by providing healthcare professionals with the most current and accurate information available.

It can also help reduce costs and increase efficiency by streamlining the decision-making process.

Image-based and radiology diagnosis

One of the areas where machine learning excels is the analysis of image data. As you may know, image analysis is a key part of several medical specialties, such as radiology, dermatology and ophthalmology.

The practice of radiology involves reading of images generated through various techniques such as X-ray, CAT scans, PET scans, etc. These images usually contain a large proportion of the information required to arrive at a diagnosis. As these techniques have been in use for decades, there is also a comprehensive library of images that can be used to train AI algorithms, making this field one of the best candidates for implementing AI solutions. In India, several startups are already in operation to support large-scale clinical diagnoses.

Radiologist Dr Selvam Kumar* recounts, 'This was during my training years in the UK. I remember this patient who was rushed into the emergency ward with severe head and neck trauma. We had to rule out a lot of possibilities including odontoid fracture, a type of fracture in the cervical spine. These fractures are very difficult to detect on standard images. The hospital had just installed an AI based system as a pilot programme and my senior used it as a tool to detect the fracture. AI tools are more likely to see subtle variations in the image and suggest if surgery was needed. In this patient's case, thanks to the AI tool diagnosing the fracture, the attending doctors were able to take immediate action. I feel that these tools will soon be available in India too and would be a boon to our profession.'

Doctors diagnose skin lesions through visual inspection. A typical skin melanoma (skin cancer) has visual characteristics that set them apart from benign moles. This makes dermatology one of the best candidates for AI-based image diagnosis. In 2017, a team of researchers created a neural network trained on 130,000 dermatological images, which has achieved specialist-level accuracy in diagnosing skin cancers, outperforming the average dermatologist in testing.[3] The aim of the research behind this experiment is for the finalized diagnostic tool to reach mobile devices, bringing expert level dermatological diagnosis to patients worldwide.

Dr Abhilasha Karnik,* a dermatologist from Coimbatore, had this to say: 'My biggest grouse as a dermatologist is that most patients come to me only when their issues are magnified. Most people tend to ignore skin issues and this leads to chronic ailments. I attended a conference on AI in dermatology and I was blown by the advances that are emerging in the field. There are apps that you can download on your phone and use it to scan your concern area. The app then uses AI tools to analyse the images and recommends the next steps. It can also send the data to a doctor for a more accurate diagnosis. This would be such a boon to so many people who are reticent about consulting a doctor for skin issues!'

Ophthalmology is the area of medicine dealing with conditions affecting the eye. The retina, the 'screen of the eye', on which the images we see are projected is one of the critical components of the human eye. Damage to the retina, through various causes such as diabetes, glaucoma and age-related degradation, is one of the leading causes of preventable blindness worldwide.

Fundus photography, a non-invasive procedure in which a special camera is used to take photographs of the retina, is the main technique used to diagnose retinal issues.[4]

A team of researchers trained an AI model to scan fundus photographs and identify signs of diabetic retinopathy, macular oedema and other retinal conditions. The AI model could not only accurately identify retinal issues, but it could also extract even previously unknown associations between retinal image patterns and age, gender, blood pressure, smoking status and a history of cardiac issues. A similar predictive model has been approved for use in the clinical setting by the FDA in the US to predict and detect diabetic retinopathy and macular oedemas.

In India, Sankara Eye Foundation and Singapore-based Leben Care have deployed a comprehensive retina risk assessment software, Netra AI, to enable faster and more accurate detection of retinal disorders in India.[5] Diabetic retinopathy is a real threat to the increasing diabetic population in India, and there are not enough ophthalmologists to screen these cases in rural areas. This is where Netra AI comes in. By analysing images from portable, technician-operated fundus camera devices, it helps get a referable diabetic retinopathy grading via a cloud-based web portal instantaneously. The solution uses AI algorithms, developed in collaboration with leading retina experts, with a four-step deep convolutional neural network. Netra AI was validated at Sankara Eye Hospital with internal and external validation images from patients. The neural network helps detect the stage of the disease and annotate lesions based on pixel density in the fundus images.

It also helps diagnose other retinal conditions like macular degeneration and other retinal pathologies, thus reducing the screening burden on healthcare specialists. Google has also worked with Sankara Nethralaya and Aravind Eye Hospital on a similar solution. Early diagnoses help in stemming the progress of the disease and may prevent total blindness in thousands of patients.

Biomarker discovery

A biomarker is a measurable indicator of a biological situation, such as a disease or response to a particular treatment. For example, a consistently elevated blood glucose level is a biomarker that indicates the presence of diabetes. Similarly, an increased level of antibodies post-vaccination is a biomarker that proves the effectiveness of that particular vaccine.

Biomarkers play an important role in the diagnosis as well as the treatment of diseases. Advances in molecular biology technologies such as genomics (mapping the entire genome, or genetic code, of an organism) and proteomics (mapping the structure and function of all proteins in an organism) have led to the discovery of millions of quantifiable data points that could serve as biomarkers. Unfortunately, the huge volume of data these technologies produce also means that manual analysis of the data is all but impossible.

This is where AI can shine. Machine learning models have been successfully used in the past to analyse and identify various factors associated with diseases by measuring parameters like gene expression, protein abundance levels and DNA methylation. These parameters can be used to predict the status of a number of diseases, such as cancers, infectious diseases and the risk of Down's Syndrome. Many biomarker analyses conducted by AI have been found to be more accurate than those conducted by experts using conventional statistical methods. Many such tests are now FDA-approved and are used to guide diagnosis and treatment selection.

Dr Surya Rajan,* an oncologist from Pune, says, 'There are days when I hate my job and myself. Giving a cancer diagnosis, and then suggesting treatment options that may or may not work but will set the patient back by lakhs of rupees, is frustrating, to put it mildly. I am always looking for advances in the field. I believe that AI calculated biomarkers will have a great impact in the field of cancer treatment. I recently read about a biomarker identified by researchers representing Emory University, Cleveland Clinic, NYU Langone Health, Weill Cornell Medicine and more. The team trained an algorithm to comb through scans of non-small cell lung cancer tumours, looking for specific indicators of how well an individual might respond to immunotherapy treatments. This is such a breakthrough! Immunotherapy is an expensive procedure, and it works only in 50 per cent of the patients. If this AI tool can help us identify which patients are best suited for this procedure, it would save everyone so much stress!'

Clinical outcome prediction and patient monitoring

AI can be used to predict patient outcomes and identify high-risk patients. By integrating data from EHR systems, it is now possible to track and predict the prognosis of patients suffering from chronic illnesses such as TB and diabetes.

This can help clinicians develop personalized treatment plans and improve patient outcomes. Wadhwani AI, partnering with the Government of India, is working on multiple TB projects that include not just radiological tools but also prediction of risk for 'Lost to Follow Up', that is, people who don't turn up for follow-up appointments. This is important for TB as the treatment is a long process that could continue for six to nine months. Many people experience side-effects that make them drop out midway, while some drop out because they feel well and think they no longer need the medication.

Wadhwani AI is also focusing its efforts on bringing this technology to rural areas. 'To assist frontline health workers, identify underweight neonates and monitor their growth, we are developing a smartphone-based technology that provides accurate, timely, geo-tagged and tamper-proof weight estimation,' a spokesperson for Wadhwani AI said.[6]

They continued, 'Globally, 2.4 million children died in the first month of life in 2019—approximately 6,700 neonatal deaths every day. Research suggests that many of these deaths are preventable if the baby's weight can be determined in the first week after birth—an enormous problem in countries such as India where a significant number of births still take place at home, with no trained midwife or medical professional in attendance.'

Virtual nursing assistants

Virtual nursing assistants are AI-powered chatbots that can provide patients with personalized medical advice and assistance. They can help patients manage chronic conditions, such as diabetes, by providing them with reminders to take their medication and monitoring their symptoms. This can hugely improve the patient's experience and health outcomes, especially for elderly patients, reducing the frequency of hospital visits. In turn, this also reduces the burden on healthcare providers.

Dr Jagdish Surana,* who owns a thirty-bed nursing home in Lucknow, says, 'A doctor's life is tough and being a businessman and a doctor is tougher. Recruiting and retaining competent staff is a huge challenge. I adopted a medical chatbot around December 2021. There was a learning curve but my team and I soon adapted to it. Most of our patients also got comfortable typing out information on the app. Thanks to the smartphone revolution, many of them are already exposed to technology. The app is a great blessing to manage chronic ailment patients. It helps them keep track of their health goals and reminds them to exercise, stick to their diet, etc. I now recommend this app to many of my doctor friends!'

Adoption of AI Technologies in Medicine

AI technologies are being rapidly adopted in healthcare systems around the world. In India, there has been a growing interest in the use of AI to improve healthcare delivery. The Indian government has launched several initiatives to promote the adoption of AI technologies in healthcare, including the National Health Stack, which aims to create a digital health infrastructure for the country.[7]

The private sector has also been active in the adoption of these technologies in healthcare. Many hospitals and healthcare providers in India are investing in AI-powered medical devices and software. For example, the Narayana Health hospital chain has implemented an AI-powered imaging system that can detect potential abnormalities in medical images.

Challenges

While AI has shown its potential to improve healthcare delivery, the path to its widespread adoption is littered with cautionary tales.

In 2015, a sixty-six-year-old Japanese woman was diagnosed with acute myeloid leukaemia, a type of blood cancer, at the University of Tokyo's Institute of Medical Science. Her doctors began a course of chemotherapy according to the treatment protocol.

After a successful round of chemotherapy, however, the doctors realized that her recovery from post-remission therapy was unusually slow. This strongly indicated that they were looking at a completely different type of leukaemia. The treatment team decided to look at a new way of finding the missing piece of the puzzle.

Enter IBM Watson, a system that combines deep machine learning and natural language processing capabilities. Watson had previously been in the news for its appearances on the US game show Jeopardy, where it beat the top champions. However, it was now faced with a much more complex task: diagnosing a living, breathing human and recommending the best course of treatment.

According to reports, Watson cross-referenced the patient's genetic data with its own database and detected over a thousand genetic mutations in her DNA. More importantly, the AI could filter out which of the thousand were diagnostically important and not just hereditary characteristics that were unrelated to her disease. This led researchers to the correct diagnosis: a rare secondary form of leukaemia caused by myelodysplastic syndromes—a group of diseases in which the bone marrow makes too few healthy blood cells.

The most important thing was that this process took Watson a grand total of ten minutes! In the world of technology, the verdict was clear: the era of AI in medicine had arrived!

The executives at IBM, the company behind Watson, were so captivated with its potential capabilities that they blindly promoted it as the next giant leap in fields as diverse as healthcare, finance and law. While the technology showed potential, all the limitations that were pointed out were ignored. IBM promised Watson would become the last word in treating cancer and poured billions of dollars into its development without appreciating the complexity of the cancers it was expected to diagnose. The launch of Watson Health, in partnership with several prominent cancer institutes, was a failure. Physicians often found themselves wrestling with the technology rather than spending more time with patients, as was promised. In January 2022, IBM finally sold off Watson Health to a private equity fund for slightly over $1 billion, a massive loss on the investment they had made.[8]

In India, as across the world, the hurdles to AI implementation in healthcare remain acute, from both technological and social perspectives.

AI is a black box

A black box is a system which takes an input and turns it into an output without anyone knowing how it actually works. In a sense, for the majority of the population, most of modern technology is a black box. We don't really understand the internal workings of our phones, computers or televisions.

What makes AI unique in this respect, however, is that even its creators are not sure how an AI system processes data. These systems are complex and are designed to learn and process information independently. In a medical context, this means that no one can tell you with certainty what path the AI followed to reach a certain diagnosis and recommendation, not even the company that created it or the engineers who maintain it. Most physicians can tell you what steps they followed to reach a certain diagnosis, and what information led them to believe that they had the right answer. Would anyone be willing to trust an AI application that cannot explain its actions in the same way?

Integrity of data

ChatGPT and its equivalents are being touted as the next big thing in the medical field. Enthusiasts are painting a colourful picture of how it can revolutionize patient care. Some of the areas it may improve are managing remote healthcare, maintaining medical records, identifying patients for clinical trials, enhancing medical education, medication management, disease surveillance, medical writing, patient triage and more.

While this looks promising, there are some inherent drawbacks.

Chatbots can function only if they have enough data fed into them. The accuracy of this data is still a question mark. Chatbots may then end up providing misleading information to patients. ChatGPT in its current form does not necessarily provide the latest data. Another big drawback is that it does not provide sources for its answers. For all we know, the source may be a random blogpost. This compromises evidence-based treatment.

Ethical concerns

Large-scale data collection gives rise to a number of ethical, social and legal concerns. Patient data is arguably the most private kind of data there is—most Western countries like the US have stringent laws that protect the privacy of patients. As AI models need access to large amounts of extremely sensitive data like genetic information, chronic disease progression, etc., one of the biggest challenges is to keep such data anonymous and out of the reach of actors that could misuse it.

AI models have also been shown to be susceptible to bias. If the models are trained on biased data, it will result in slanted predictions and recommendations. Bias in data can be a result of bad sampling practices, leading to the overrepresentation or the exclusion of a particular group, be it ethnic, demographic or racial. Reducing bias is one of the key steps in obtaining high-quality training data.

Lack of data

AI development and implementation is extremely costly, and one of the most expensive steps in the process is the collection and processing of training data used to teach its models. Raw data is often unstructured, containing millions of irrelevant data points, and needs to undergo extensive cleaning and processing before it can be fed to the AI algorithm.

One of the main limitations of AI in medicine is the lack of high-quality data. As a safety-critical application with almost no margin for error, AI models deployed in healthcare need to get the result right the first time. If these algorithms are trained on poor-quality data, their predictions will likely be wrong.

Moreover, due to differences in demographics, the data needs to be as specific to the region as possible. It would be erroneous to use medical data gathered in an urban area of the US such as New York as a baseline to make predictions about patients in rural Uttar Pradesh. The two populations could hardly be more different in terms of genetics, lifestyle and food habits.

In India, medical data collection remains primitive. Records are often incomplete, inconsistent or of poor quality. Most rural health centres barely maintain any records at all, and those that do still mostly rely on pen and paper. The huge variation in lifestyles and diets within India itself makes insights derived from data collected in one part of India not always fully applicable to patients in another part. While it is possible to put systems in place today to begin collecting relevant data more effectively, it will take years before these efforts bear fruit, not to mention the huge financial investment this would incur. The fact remains that without such investments, AI cannot be relied on to get everything right.

Lack of lateral thinking

One of AI's limitations is an inability to look beyond the given or available data. While AI can far exceed humans in analysing vast amounts of data and identifying patterns in them, it is still not always capable of synthesizing hypotheses of its own, to think outside the box, the way highly experienced clinicians can. How often is this needed is another question altogether, but this still remains an area where AI has to catch up.

Says Dr Mridula Pandit,* an internist with over thirty-five years of experience treating patients in a clinical setting, 'Over the years, I have realized that 80 per cent of my job is to simply provide a listening ear to the patient. If you carefully listen to them and ask the right questions to guide the conversation, the patient themselves will tell you everything you need to know to make the right diagnosis. The true skill of a physician is to gather and synthesize a diagnosis from what a patient tells you, combining it with your own observations, test results and other tools. Often, you will find that the actual problem the patient suffers from is completely different to the symptoms that they present at the beginning of the consultation. You need to be a good listener and a detective. It's all in the communication skills.'

AI will surely get better in the years to come but, at the moment, it does have difficulty 'listening' and interpreting what is not already present in the data it works with.

Cost factor

Developing, deploying and maintaining an AI system is currently expensive. It requires the work of a large number of specialists with new skillsets. AI systems are also extremely processor-intensive, requiring the use of powerful new chips with plenty of storage and high-power consumption. In a country like India, where public spending on healthcare remains at a paltry 2.1 per cent of GDP in 2023, there is a lot of investment required in order to put both the infrastructure and skill in place to take advantage of the possibilities that AI brings to the table. Unless the government aggressively raises healthcare spending and significantly invests in developing AI infrastructure, the pace of adoption will likely remain slow. Of course, if the private sector sees revenue opportunities in using AI, they can make this transition happen much faster, perhaps as soon as the end of the current decade.

Cultural resistance to change

Healthcare is an industry that is notoriously embedded in its age-old practices, with an established pattern of working, a clearly defined hierarchy and its own code of behaviour. Introducing a technology as revolutionary as AI risks disrupting the existing order and will draw a lot of resistance.

Physicians trust themselves to get a diagnosis right and will not relish delegating the task of making crucial diagnostic decisions to AI. It will take a lot of effort and training to get physicians comfortable with using the technology and seeing it as a powerful new tool in their arsenal rather than a mindless replacement for hard-earned skills perfected over years of practice.

An alternative approach would be to build a new healthcare model from the ground, where AI is integrated into the workflow from the very beginning for handling the more basic administrative and data processing tasks, as well as in primary diagnostics, while the physician is free to focus on providing high-touch, personalized treatment to the patient.

Accountability

Accountability is also an important factor. If a doctor misdiagnoses a patient, they can be held responsible under malpractice laws. But what happens when an AI software gives a wrong recommendation? Who will be held liable? Will it be the administrators of the hospital or the company that implemented the AI or the engineers who built the model or the data scientists who created the training data? A proper chain of accountability should be established to address mistakes and malfunctions and get rid of this legal grey area before AI can be brought into the mainstream use.

Need for a new regulatory framework

Governments over the world have had a poor track record in regulating high-tech industries. However, without putting such a framework in place, deploying AI can lead to a free-for-all that could affect the patient and degrade the healthcare experience of millions.

A comprehensive approach that takes into account the legal, ethical and social aspects should be brought in to regulate the deployment of AI systems in healthcare. This new framework should enshrine protections for patients' privacy, establish a clear pathway for accountability in case of failure and provide guidelines to eliminate biases in data used by AI. Creating this will be a complicated and arduous process but it is absolutely essential if India is to ride the wave of the fast-approaching revolution in AI.

Infrastructure and connectivity

India still struggles with healthcare infrastructure and connectivity, particularly in rural areas. The implementation of AI-powered medical systems requires high-speed internet connectivity, which is not always available in many parts of the country. While India has seen great progress in mobile phone connectivity using 4G networks over the past decade, with a phenomenal growth in subscribers, the infrastructure that enables these networks to operate remains patchy in rural areas. Without reliable high-speed connections, it will be difficult to realize the potential of AI in underserved areas. The arrival of the next wave of connectivity technology such as 5G, if implemented with maximum coverage in mind, should mitigate this challenge significantly.

Final Thoughts

Whether we like it or not, progress cannot be reversed, and AI is here to stay. While most of its applications are still in the early stages of development, there is no doubt that by the 2030s, the way the healthcare industry functions will have changed dramatically.

India, with all its special challenges, will not lag behind in the AI revolution. I believe that AI has the potential to completely transform healthcare delivery in the country.

AI has the promise to become the single biggest gamechanger in healthcare, rivalling even the discovery of antibiotics or insulin. Sooner than later, I foresee companies emerging that can bring AI-based diagnostics to the patient directly. While such a model carries obvious risks, any company that dares to take the plunge could change the world of healthcare, causing disruption on an unprecedented scale. Imagine diagnosing and treating yourself, never having to leave home to visit the doctor! If I was a betting man (sadly, I am not), I would be willing to put down a lot of money on this happening in the next fifteen years.

13

A Doctor's Dilemma

In June 2019, a seventy-five-year-old male patient passed away at the government-run Nil Ratan Sircar (NRS) Medical College and Hospital in Kolkata. The family of the deceased was duly notified and by 11 p.m., a group of family members arrived at the hospital. They concluded that the death was due to alleged negligence by the medical team and instead of raising a complaint and seeking an enquiry, they did what a mob does best when emotions run amok. They became violent and turned the hospital premises into a battleground. The staff members, including two intern doctors, were injured in the clash. One of the interns, Dr Paribaha Mukhopadhyay, suffered a skull fracture after a brick hit his head. He had to undergo multiple surgeries over the next few months and developed sores on his tongue due to the medications. Between surgeries, he was advised to rest and reduce stress. He was lucky that he did not have any lasting brain injury that may have left him incapable of working, or worse.

Following this attack, a group of his colleagues shut the gates of the hospital as a protest and demanded security for the staff. The protest spread to other hospitals as other doctors were also concerned about their safety. As junior doctors of Burdwan Medical College and Hospital were protesting at the hospital's emergency gate, a mob of relatives of patients hurled bricks at them, injuring three junior doctors and a fourth-year student, Mayank Agarwal, suffered serious eye injuries as a result.

As always when doctors protest, there was a public outcry condemning the protests. Political parties also jumped in, and the main issue was soon sidetracked. Eventually, the doctors called off the protests and resumed work.

The police had arrested a few people from the original mob that attacked Dr Paribaha Mukhopadhyay but they were soon released on bail.[1] Given the state of our judicial system, it is anybody's guess as to when or if justice would finally prevail!

Stories about irate mobs beating up doctors and healthcare providers abound. People also bash up doctors and nurses on social media. Why do people forget that healthcare providers are human too? In India, the struggle to become a doctor starts at an absurdly young age. Students put their lives on hold to follow this path and it is a long, arduous journey before they make any money at all.

The aim of this book is not to bash the healthcare provider community or to highlight its failings. Healthcare providers face various challenges that impede them from delivering optimum care, and this aspect needs to be given careful consideration in the context of all that we have seen in the previous chapters.

In this chapter, we will explore some of the challenges healthcare providers face in their efforts to deliver optimum care. In some ways, this is the chapter that I hope will redeem me to some extent from the wrath of my colleagues who read this book!

Becoming a Doctor

Let us start at the very beginning: gaining admission into a medical college. Even in my days, it was not easy to get a seat in a medical college. Today, it is a Herculean task.

In March 2023, the Minister of State in the Ministry of Health and Family Welfare, Bharati Pravin Pawar, informed the Parliament that there are 660 medical colleges providing 1,01,043 MBBS seats as of date. Out of these, 52,778 are available in government medical colleges and the remaining 48,265 seats are in the private sector.[2]

How does one get admission into these colleges? Through the National Eligibility cum Entrance Test (NEET), a single entrance test for admissions to MBBS and BDS in colleges across India. It received a record breaking 20.8 lakh applications in 2023! Not all of them would clear the exam, though. In 2021, 16 lakh candidates took the exam, and about 8 lakh aspirants cleared the test.[3] These 8 lakh students vied for the then available 80,000 seats—so only 10 per cent of the candidates finally got admission into a medical college. The NEET is not without controversy and the MCI has been accused of pushing it down the throats of hapless students. Some have also alleged that it is biased towards the privileged and is anti-poor. While there may be a change in the selection process in the future, NEET remains the single point for admission into an MBBS college.

Sushant Kelkar* recounts, 'I come from a middle-class family. My father works as an accountant in a private firm and my mother is a primary school teacher in a government school. I'm the eldest of three children. Our parents have always insisted on academic intelligence, and my siblings and I were always class toppers. My father had aspired to become a doctor but he could not as he was forced to start working at a young age after the untimely demise of his father. From a very young age, I had been told that it is my duty to fulfil his dreams. As a child, I had no idea about a career, and I promised that I would become a doctor. My parents did a lot of research and enrolled me in coaching classes from the time I was in Class 8. I was not allowed to have any hobbies. They ensured that I spent every moment out of school preparing for the entrance exam. The coaching fees was not cheap, and I noticed that my mother took to wearing glass bangles by the time I was in the twelfth standard. I finally appeared for the NEET exam in 2019. Frankly, I was exhausted with the preparations.

I had no life outside studies. I had no friends and no one who I could talk to about my frustrations. My father would keep reminding me that this was a do-or-die exam and he depended on me to get into MBBS. By February 2019, I started having nightmares about failing the exam, thus disappointing my parents. I would wake up, drenched in sweat, and couldn't go back to sleep. I would anyway start my day at 5 a.m. so that I could attend the coaching class at 6 a.m. On the day of the exam, I just blanked out and couldn't remember anything. The questions on the paper seemed to be in an alien language and I couldn't answer a single question. I was so scared that I slipped away from the test centre and ran away to the railway station. I would have got onto a train if it was not for my uncle, my mother's brother, who saw me at the station. He took me back home and when I told my parents what happened, my father removed his belt and started hitting me. My mother did not stop him but my uncle intervened and suggested that I go to his house till my father cools down. It has been three years, and my father has not spoken a word to me. I joined a graduate course and stared earning a living by giving tuitions. I don't know what the future has in store for me.'

Sushant's case is just one among thousands. Not all NEET aspirants are self-motivated. Many are pushed by their parents and forced to attend expensive coaching courses. A coaching course can set one back by almost ₹1.5 lakhs for a two-year programme. The higher the brand's reputation, the higher the cost.

Medical education is not cheap; it can range from ₹20,000 to ₹7.5 lakhs in a government college and from ₹20 lakh to more than a crore in a private college. This is for the five-and-a-half-year MBBS course (four-and-a-half years of classes plus one year of internship). How many students can afford this? Nayana Reddy relates, 'I come from a low-income family. I have always dreamed of becoming a doctor and my parents supported me completely. I worked very hard through my school years and got a scholarship for NEET coaching. I cleared the exam with 520 marks, which was okay but not enough to get admission into a government college. I secured admission in a private college, where the fees were around ₹75 lakhs. My father is the sole breadwinner of the family, and he earns around ₹7 lakhs a year. He refused to give up. He sold the little bit of land we had and my mother's jewellery and borrowed the rest from various people. He took on an additional job as a night security guard to add to his earnings. I am now in my final year but I know the sacrifices my family has made for my education. I still have many years to go before I can start earning a decent income. If I had known that life would be so tough, I would not have chosen this profession.'

A final-year MBBS student Naveen Kumar Kadkol died by suicide a week before his convocation.[4] A hardworking student, he was to graduate from one of the top-ranked medical colleges in the country. In his note, he stated that he suffered from social anxiety. Many MBBS students we spoke to also stated that they were extremely stressed and anxious. Pariniti Mukhopadhyay,* a twenty-three-year-old MBBS student, says, 'Getting into a medical college is tough. Most of us have worked hard to get into the college, and in that process, have a limited or no social life. Though I have always wanted to become a doctor, I was not ready for the stark reality. Seeing so much illness and realizing that I would be responsible for curing them—it was harrowing! I don't have anyone to talk to about all these as my parents are not from the field. Some of my friends even talk about ending their lives and sometimes I find myself agreeing with them. But somehow, I find the strength to carry on. In the three years I have been in this college, there have already been two deaths by suicide and seven students have dropped out across the years due to the stress.'

An MBBS degree is not enough to make a decent living as a doctor. A postgraduate degree is essential. There are around 42,182 PG seats including seats for Doctor of Medicine (MD), Master of Surgery (MS) and diploma courses.[5] Depending on the specialization and the college, the course can set a student back by ₹10 lakhs to ₹2 crores and upwards. Many students prefer to go outside the country for their postgraduation as the costs are much lesser and they feel that the quality of education is better. With so many challenges and such a large financial commitment, is it any wonder that many doctors have an 'earn as much as possible' outlook rather than an altruistic one?

A Doctor's Life

An individual becomes an MBBS doctor after five-and-a-half years of studies and internship. Often, students prefer to work for a couple of years before pursuing a postgraduate degree, mainly for financial reasons. A PG degree takes three years, while a diploma takes two, depending on the specialization. By the time many doctors are done with their PG, they are in their late twenties or early thirties. After this, some will go on to get a super specialty degree. As we have seen, not everyone gets a high-paying job immediately. Many doctors spend their initial years earning a paltry salary which is not commensurate with their expertise. A government doctor can be posted anywhere across the state—sometimes at places with frequent power cuts, inadequate running water or even proper sanitation facilities. Doctors consult an enormous number of patients every day and hence are also prone to infections and are even at risk of contracting diseases like TB and COVID-19 from patients. Many rural areas do not even have adequate running water to wash hands between patients, leaving the doctors vulnerable to infections.

Doctors have long working hours, especially during their internships and initial years. Thirty-six-hour shifts are common. They survive on greasy cafeteria food and quick naps between patients. Is it any wonder that doctors often feel the effects of burn out even before they enter the job market?

Continuous education is a must and even senior doctors spend a lot of time updating their knowledge. Today, there is the additional challenge of learning new techniques and technologies in a rapidly changing field.

Clearly, this is not something that is easy for everyone. Doctors have challenges that exceed most other professions.

For doctors in India, balancing their family and social life and career is an everyday battle, no matter where they are in their career.

Pay structure

The popularly held belief is that medicine is one of the best paid and prestigious professions. While the prestige associated with being a doctor is undeniable, the pay is disproportionately lower, especially after taking into account the gruelling training and hectic lifestyle. 'Most doctors make very little money at the beginning of their careers,' says Dr Nirmal Mohanty,* a professor at one of the top medical schools. 'It is only maybe fifteen years into their careers that doctors' pay starts to catch up to those of other professionals such as engineers or lawyers. A fresh graduate with an MBBS degree is often offered an insultingly low salary. For comparison, a delivery rider working for one of these food delivery startups can easily make more than a junior doctor who puts in eighteen-hour shifts on the regular. Everything about this life is exhausting, and we're not even paid well for it. But the popular perception of the rich doctor is shaped by the top 1 per cent of doctors who have specializations in very glamorous, niche or in-demand fields. Looking at these doctors and assuming that the average doctor makes that kind of money is, frankly, laughable.'

A doctor's life is not just demanding physically, but also is emotionally sapping. It is not easy to face life-and-death situations every day. Dr Mohanty comments, 'A twenty-four- or twenty-five-year-old doctor is expected to have the emotional maturity to manage themselves and the relatives when a patient cannot be saved. Most of the time, the doctor does not even have the luxury of taking a few moments to grieve as there is always another patient who needs attention.'

Another issue is how medical degrees from India are valued. After facing the brutal competition of getting through the graduate and postgraduate medical entrance exams, many doctors find themselves stuck in the Indian job market. 'While our skills are on par with, and our training as intense, if not more so, as doctors in the West, the value of our degrees could not be more different,' says Dr Bindu Panicker,* a specialist physician based out of Visakhapatnam. She recounts, 'Early in my career, a couple of years after my MD, I moved to my first job at a well-known corporate hospital, with a decent bump in pay. A couple of weeks later, they hired another doctor, a fresh MD graduate, who was being paid almost twice as much as I was. The reason? She had a degree from the US. With my degree, it is almost impossible to practice outside of India without going through a long, laborious process of recertification and licensing. But someone who had studied in the West would be welcomed back with a red carpet. I felt I had made a huge mistake putting myself through the whole process of getting an MD in India. Had I studied in the West, in the UK or the US, I would've had a much greater range of options to choose from and higher earnings to offset the increased cost. Was it even worth it?'

We can see how this line of reasoning can quickly become a huge problem in India, when retaining our medical talent is challenging enough already. The rate of brain drain can accelerate exponentially if the system doesn't value the ones who are critical to its functioning.

Violence against doctors

Violence against doctors is not a new phenomenon and is not restricted to India. In China, a dentist was killed by an aggrieved patient—twenty years after the treatment—indicating that it was not spur-of-the-moment rage but calculated and cold-blooded murder.[6] In Western countries, cases of violence have been reported during house visits, especially night-time, waiting areas in clinics, psychiatric wards, emergency rooms, paediatric wards and ICUs. The perpetrators can either be the patient or family and friends of the patient.

In India, the patient is rarely the perpetrator. Relatives, neighbours, local goons, even political forces and sometimes random bystanders who have absolutely no connection with the patient, jump into the fray.

A few major incidents of violence against doctors in India:[7]

- 14 June 2019: A doctor was tied to a tree, robbed of his money and belongings; his wife and daughter were gang raped in the Gaya district of Bihar.

- 1 January 2019: A senior paediatrician was brutally assaulted by the patient's family at his clinic in Himayatnagar, Hyderabad, Telangana.
- 15 October 2018: The relatives of a patient assaulted a doctor from the reserved category demanding the service of an upper-class doctor at Jabalpur, Madhya Pradesh.
- 19 May 2018: A patient's relative beat up two resident doctors of J.J. Hospital, Mumbai.
- 15 March 2017: An orthopaedic doctor at a government hospital in Dhule, Maharashtra, who was brutally assaulted by a patient's kin, developed blurring of vision in one eye.

The country also witnessed many acts of violence against doctors and the nursing staff during the peak of the COVID-19 pandemic. Doctors were asked to move houses or were beaten up, mobs blocked funerals of doctors—the list goes on.

While I understand that the families of the patient are anxious and are overcome with grief when a loved one dies, is it really fair to attack the doctor? Often, the reason cited is suspicion of wrongdoing by the doctors or inadequate care given to the patient or delays in treatments. Walk into a government hospital and the first thing you notice is the teeming crowd of people. Wards are full and emergency rooms are stretched to their limits. The number of doctors is not proportionate to the number of patients. Often, doctors have been working on twenty-four-hour-shifts and are exhausted not just with fatigue, but also with the stress of caring for so many people. No doctor likes to be the harbinger of bad news but they cannot save all the people under their care. It is frightening to be at the receiving end of an angry, uncontrollable mob.

Dr Gaurishankar Biswas,* a researcher with a pharmaceutical company, shares his story, 'I was working as a GP in a small town in Bihar. I had my own clinic and, apart from a compounder cum receptionist, did not have any other employee. I had a thriving practice. I used to open my clinic at 9 a.m. and would continue to see patients till 8 p.m., though the official closing time was 5 p.m. I would gulp down some food whenever I found a few minutes in the day. It was not as if I was making a lot of money as my charges were nominal and many patients would promise to pay later. One evening, just as I was closing the clinic, a vehicle screeched to a halt, and I heard a commotion outside. I turned around and saw six or seven people jump from a jeep, dragging a man who was visibly injured. I rushed to him and noticed a bullet wound on his stomach and he had lost a lot of blood. When I checked his pulse, it was very thready. I knew that I could not save him—he needed surgery, and my clinic was not equipped for it. I told the accompanying people to rush him to the private hospital which was around a kilometre away from my clinic. They did not listen and insisted that I treat him. I tried explaining to them that time was of the essence and that my clinic was not adequately equipped and that I was willing to accompany them to the hospital. They did not listen and started hurling abuses at me. In the mayhem, the patient died. After I declared him dead, one of them pushed me down to the ground. The others started kicking me and spitting at me. One of them even urinated on me. Though there was a crowd of people who gathered, no one did anything to help me. The gang sped away when the police arrived. The police rushed me to the hospital where I was diagnosed with multiple fractures—on my left leg, my ribs and my right wrist. It was sheer agony. I was in the hospital for weeks and had to undergo intensive rehabilitation post-discharge. I was wheelchair bound for months. I was in my mid-thirties then and did not have a lot of savings. The medical expenses were very high, and my wife's family sold their land to help us meet these expenses. I later learned that the wounded person was the son of an influential local politician and goon. The police who were supposed to protect me threatened me with dire consequences if I filed a formal police complaint. The goon's henchmen made a similar threat to my wife. None of the witnesses were willing to come forward in my defence. Is this why I became a doctor? Do you know how many people I have treated and how many lives I have saved? After a lot of thought, I moved out of that town. I was so disheartened that I just could not practice medicine any longer. I came to Mumbai and got a job in a pharmaceutical company as a researcher. I do not have any interactions with the public and I have saner work timings and yes, I earn better. I still suffer from post-traumatic stress disorder (PTSD), panic attacks and I am under medication and go for therapy. The other day, when my eight-year-old son announced that he wanted to become a doctor, I sat him down and dissuaded him. I, who was such an idealist!' he ends with a sigh.

Electronic and social media are not the judge and jury. It is the responsibility of the hospital and the courts to discipline the doctor if they're found guilty after a thorough investigation. In recent years, political parties have been quick to jump into the fray without bothering to find the truth.

When doctors protest against violence, there is a hue and cry. Are doctors supposed to serve the people at the cost of their lives? They do that anyway, as was seen in the recent pandemic. The medical fraternity worked tirelessly against an unknown disease.

Unless the central and state governments take strict action against perpetuators, doctors will not feel safe.

Doctor or employee?

The prestige of being attached to a corporate hospital is a status symbol that few doctors can resist. Disillusioned with government hospitals, more and more people are choosing to work for the private sector. Corporate hospitals have been swallowing up smaller clinics and nursing homes, leaving patients with few options. The marketing blitz by these hospitals have convinced the public that these hospitals offer the best treatment and have the best doctors. These hospitals also aggressively recruit doctors.

Dr Sudeep Belagavi,* an orthopaedic surgeon based out of Mysore, says, 'I had my own clinic in Mysore and had a busy practice. I had a tie-up with a local hospital for conducting surgeries. My job was not just limited to seeing patients, but I also had to manage payments, vendor management, clinic management, etc. It was also difficult for me to close my clinic if I took a vacation. I was thirty-eight and had paid off my loans but had almost no savings. My children were growing, and I had to start saving for their education. It was then that the local hospital was taken over by a famous corporate chain. They made me an offer to join them as the head of orthopaedics. The salary was very attractive, and I would be managing a team. It was an offer I could not refuse. After a few months of working, I was given a target to achieve. As the weeks passed, the pressure to contribute increased and I started with an unnecessary surgery that would bring in revenue. I also started recommending expensive tests for patients. Patient care is still the cornerstone of my practice, but what is the harm if I make some much-needed money in the process?'

Often, infrastructure and equipment procured at great cost by the hospital has to be put to use, regardless of whether it is required for the patients or not. The doctor becomes a pawn in the entire system, with the only option available being to play along or quit the hospital. And going to the next hospital will not provide any respite either as the situation is very likely to be the same.

Temptations

Sanjay Maurya,* a sales manager with a top multinational pharmaceutical company, says, 'We have instructions from our bosses to increase the sales of a few of our premium brands. Our brands are priced higher than generics though they don't really differ from generics. We convince doctors by offering them commissions to prescribe our brands. The commission can range from 15 per cent to 40 per cent, depending on the city and the reputation of the doctor. The money is deposited into accounts of their choice. We also offer a lot of other freebies—all-expenses-paid conferences at foreign locales where they can take their family too, expensive gadgets, cash, gold, etc. It is not just us who are doing it. Haven't you read media reports about how the manufacturers of Dolo-650 allegedly spent ₹1,000 crores on sales promotion?'

This industry is notorious for corrupting doctors the world over, offering them everything from supermarket and fuel coupons to exotic foreign trips in return for prescriptions of their drugs. Doctors often find it difficult to resist such temptations. Lax regulation of the pharma industry is also to blame.

The phenomenon of kickbacks from lab and radiology centres continues to this day, though of late, there have been attempts to discourage this illegal practice. Doctors can get as much as ₹5,000 for prescribing a single MRI scan and almost always this amount is door delivered in cash to the doctor. The practice of kickbacks from labs and radiology centres thrives both in metro cities and in semi-urban centres despite medical associations asking their members to desist from this practice and the government declaring it illegal.

Not all doctors fall prey to these tactics, but it would require superhuman effort to resist these temptations. It is a myth that all doctors are rich and don't need the money.

Working hours

Except in some specialties, doctors do not really have fixed working hours. The hours of practice may be defined but there will always be the need to attend to patients who call or visit outside official working hours. In their initial years, doctors work long shifts, often for periods longer than twenty-four hours at a stretch. No one realizes the toll such long hours of work running into years takes on the body and mind of the doctor. If factory workers are asked to work a few hours longer, the worker's unions raise a hue and cry. But doctors and nurses do not have anyone to plead their cause.

It is not just doctors who pay the price. Even their families and friends are accustomed to last-minute cancellations if there is an emergency for a patient. Dr Gavin Barucha,* a GP based out of Colaba, Mumbai, says, 'It was my daughter's school annual day function, and she had the lead role in a play. I had promised her that I would be there. It was a proud moment for me as a father. As I was leaving the clinic, a patient arrived. He was complaining of chest pain and so I simply had to see him. It took a good thirty minutes to get his ECG and a Troponin test and to give him an all-clear and another few minutes to give him a prescription. By the time I left the clinic, around forty-five minutes later, it was closer to the evening rush hour and by the time I reached the school, my daughter's play was over. My daughter was very hurt, and my wife and daughter did not speak to me for a week!'

Doesn't a doctor deserve a family and social life? For the public these are occupational hazards, part of the job of being a doctor, and they are right to a point. But society does need to understand and appreciate that the life of a doctor is not easy. Many sacrifices are called for and made over the duration of a career.

Continuous learning

As I have mentioned in the earlier chapters, there are few other fields that require so much constant learning. Today's doctors need to know medicine, the latest developments in their field, technology, patient management, basic administration, counselling techniques, etc. And remember, they have the same twenty-four hours in a day as everyone else.

Staying abreast of the latest developments requires a lot of studying, poring over research and judging the veracity of the various publications.

I know many people outside the medical field who announce that technology is not their cup of tea. I have a few friends who still prefer dealing in cash rather than use UPI payments. But can a doctor get away today with a similar announcement? Right from video consultations to online prescriptions to using AI applications for treatment, technology is everywhere. The learning curve is quite steep for many doctors. But still, they have to persist if they want to stay relevant.

The Google/WhatsApp medical school graduates

The pandemic witnessed the sprouting of a new medical school: The WhatsApp School of Medicine. For over a decade now, the Google School of Medicine has also been witnessing astounding growth. Neither school has a strict admission policy. Anyone with a device and access to the internet can get admission for the cost of a device and connectivity.

Anand Sukumar,* a fifty-year-old technology leader recalls, 'In December 2020, my father who lives alone in Chennai contracted COVID-19 and was admitted to the hospital. Luckily, he had mild symptoms, but we were worried as he had other comorbidities. On the fifth day, I got an indignant call from him complaining that the doctors were not listening to him. Apparently, there were some specific herbs that help cure COVID-19 and the hospital was refusing to give it to him. What were his sources? WhatsApp messages from his friends and acquaintances. I tried telling him that he is in a hospital and the doctors know better than his friends, and that if indeed there were these herbs, the whole world wouldn't be suffering, but he was not convinced! Even after his discharge, he ranted about how those herbs could have helped him better.'

The doctor of today is confronted by a much more aware and well-informed patient than was the case twenty-five years ago. While greater patient awareness is welcome, the constant second-guessing of the doctor's treatment options with information obtained from the Google School of Medicine is grating. The school offers diagnosis, alternate diagnoses, treatment recommendations and side-effects of treatments. I constantly have patients call me an hour or two after they have bought the medicine I have prescribed saying that a Google search on the prescribed medicine revealed serious side-effects. It takes a great deal of patience to tell several patients a day that I am aware of those effects and they are extremely rare and are extremely unlikely to occur in this patient. Increasingly, there are patients who walk in with a self-made diagnosis and order the treatment they think I should give them. A Google search on any symptom invariably lists cancer as one of the possibilities and today's doctors first have to calm down the patients even before they start the diagnostic process!

Even worse are patients who want my opinion on alternative treatments that are supposedly free of side-effects. Dr Mangesh Kumar,* a rheumatologist based out of Gurgaon, says, 'The minute I diagnose a patient with rheumatoid arthritis and prescribe medicines, they start asking me about Ayurvedic treatments. I am an allopathic doctor and do not have knowledge of Ayurveda.

In my experience, adjunct therapies like physiotherapy, psychotherapy, etc., do help together, with the relevant allopathic medicines. Often, patients would stop the prescribed treatment and seek alternatives suggested by their friends and come back to me in a worse state of health. These are educated people! I understand that desperation pushes people to try all alternatives but, for heaven's sake, check with me before you stop the treatment. I am here to help. These are the same patients who then go around bad-mouthing me. It is a no-win situation!'

Doctors have to take all this in their stride and remain cheerful, composed and compassionate even when at times they may feel like strangling the inconsiderate and boorish patient or relative!

Remember, Doctors Are Humans Too!

It is very well to say doctors should be true to the Hippocratic oath and desist from practices that deviate from their oath. But in the times of Hippocrates, medical education did not cost a fortune. Doctors neither had huge education loans nor the sword of EMIs dangling over their heads.

This is not to justify their actions but to merely state that doctors are not some special noble species over and above those in other professions. They too have needs and have the same ethics as other professionals in society. This argument that practising medicine is a noble profession and must therefore not be placed on the same pedestal as, say, law was a proposition that ended decades ago.

Patients have become increasingly aware, demanding and aggressive, and this leads to doctors having to practise defensive medicine by ordering more tests and ensuring that they are not putting themselves at any risk of either a legal problem or, worse, being beaten up, as is increasingly happening across the country.

Doctors work long hours and put in enormous efforts, sacrificing family and personal time. While many of them are driven by a passion for the work they do and the desire to heal, the rotten apples in the profession are giving them a bad name.

Doctors achieve their peak earning potential later than other professionals do. By the time a doctor starts to earn a decent amount of money they are already in their forties with over fifteen years of experience. Pay scales in the first decade after qualification are pitiful and it is common for doctors in their mid or late thirties to compare themselves with software professionals in their mid-twenties and lament their fate.

Stringent regulation helps cut down malpractice. The fact that India has an almost unregulated healthcare industry means that healthcare providers often get away with a lot more than they can in the developed world. Human nature being what it is, more hospitals and doctors tend to take advantage of a lax system.

There are thousands of outstanding doctors in the system in India, staying true to the oath they have taken to maintain medicine and healthcare as a noble profession. But, increasingly, they are pushed into a corner where they are forced to compromise their core values and turn their back on a patient-centric approach.

It is the responsibility of society, and especially the government, to create the environment that enables doctors to earn a decent living while practising ethical medicine. Better regulation of the healthcare industry will go a long way towards making this happen.

14
Navigating the Indian Healthcare System

- How do you choose a good doctor?
- How do you select a hospital for inpatient treatment?

I have collated a few points that may help you take these crucial decisions. Apart from this, I have also listed some factors that we, as doctors, expect from patients.

Get Good Health Insurance

The first all-important thing you should do is get health insurance. I cannot stress this point enough. Being uninsured can spell financial ruin even for a well-to-do family.

At the very least, choose a basic package that will cover up to, say, ₹5 lakhs with one insurance company. Then choose a top-up policy for coverage from, say, ₹5–25 lakhs with a different company for higher coverage.

If you take away just one point from this book, let it be this: GET HEALTH INSURANCE.

How Do You Choose a Good Doctor?

Selecting a doctor is by no means an easy task. At present, most of us go by word of mouth, using references from relatives or neighbours or friends or choosing a place close to our residence. Today, many of us also check online reviews. Be aware that online reviews cannot be completely relied upon as they can be manipulated.

> Ask these questions while selecting a doctor – be it a GP or a specialist. If most of these can be answered with a 'yes', then you are most likely in good hands.
>
> - Does the doctor have a postgraduate degree? While doctors with just an MBBS are qualified and highly capable (especially some of the older doctors), a postgraduate degree does ensure a higher level of knowledge. A specialist *must* have additional qualifications in that specific area.
> - Is the doctor over the age of thirty-five? Younger doctors, while capable, might not have the depth of experience that a senior doctor would have.
> - Is the doctor attached to a hospital? Large hospitals tend to do their due diligence, so you

can be assured of the veracity of the doctor's qualifications. Also, these doctors tend to have more patients and hence more exposure.

- Is the doctor available for a consultation within a reasonable time frame? You need a doctor to be available when you have a problem and not have to wait for a week or more just for an appointment.

- Is the doctor's clinic clean and hygienic? Do the nurse or attendant follow the proper processes for a triage?

- Is the doctor an empathetic and engaged listener and communicator? Do they answer all your questions and doubts clearly?

- Is the doctor okay with getting the prescriptions filled and tests done at a place of your choice and convenience? If the doctor insists on you going to a particular pharmacy or lab, that is a red flag.

- Is the doctor's first prescription a relatively short list? Unless you have a particularly serious health issue, for most other cases, a maximum of two or three medicines would suffice.

- Is the doctor as engaged and responsive during review and subsequent visits? A doctor showing progressively lesser interest during follow-up visits is often a warning sign.

- Is the doctor available in case there is an emergency? In today's connected world, some

> doctors share their numbers or email ids for emergency purposes. Ensure that you have either of these contact details with you at all times. In case the doctor is not sharing their details, ask for the details of their secretary or assistant. But remember that these are to be used only if there is an emergency. For all non-emergency situations send them a text and do not call. Respect their boundaries at all times. If there is a serious emergency, go to the nearest hospital immediately instead of waiting for your doctor to respond.

How Do You Select a Hospital for Inpatient Treatment?

Here are a few things to keep in mind while selecting a hospital:

> - Ensure that the hospital is certified by the NABH. Similarly, for labs, check for NABL accreditation. This assures you that a third party has ascertained that the hospital has the infrastructure and capability to deliver good care.
> - Learn what people who have used the hospital's services have to say about it. Again, be wary of only relying on online reviews. Also, do not get influenced by the hospital's appearance.

- If your doctor practises in a hospital with bad reviews, check with the doctor to see if they work with any other hospital.
- Ensure that the hospital is within a twenty-minute drive from your home. Often, hospital stays require almost daily visits to the hospital and distance may add to the stress.
- Check if the hospital you choose takes your insurance, preferably in a cashless mode.
- Check that the hospital is clean and well-maintained, and the doctors and staff practice adequate hygiene measures. This goes a long way in reducing the possibility of HAIs.

How to Be a Proactive Patient

Remember that an alert and proactive patient and family can save as many lives in a hospital as the doctors can. Here's what you can do to make the most of the healthcare system:

- Ask questions at every stage. DO NOT feel that the doctor or nurse will get annoyed. It is much better to have a healthy patient and an annoyed doctor than a happy doctor with a very sick patient only because you were diffident. You can politely clarify your doubts and always ask questions that you feel you need answers to.

- Before undergoing a major surgery or procedure, always get a second opinion from another doctor at a different hospital. This will help in learning all the options available to you and the risks involved before arriving at an informed decision.
- At every stage in the hospital, let the staff know if you or the patient you are accompanying develops fresh symptoms or sense something amiss. Do not expect the hospital staff to pick up on such changes early. When at the bedside of the patient, look for any changes in their alertness level, their comfort or any alarms that may be going off from the monitors.
- If hospitalized and given the option of a discharge, take it at the first available opportunity. Hospitals are dangerous places, and you should not stay there one moment longer than absolutely necessary.
- If you perceive any deficiencies in the service provided, point them out politely. You are not the only patient in the hospital and sometimes, the staff may have overlooked something.
- You are entitled to receive your entire case record when you leave the hospital. That includes all your lab reports and images and CDs of radiology tests. Insist on digital or physical copies as applicable.

Remember Your Responsibilities

As a patient or caregiver, you are entitled to your rights. But you also have responsibilities. Being aware of these will make the process of healthcare delivery smoother for both parties.

- Once you have chosen your doctor, you need to work in tandem with them and give them your trust, while being alert at all times.
- Always be polite in your interactions with doctors and the staff. Do not raise your voice or threaten the staff, no matter how stressed you may be.
- A well-prepared patient is always easier to treat. Jot down your complaints before you visit the doctor. Take all your medical records and current list of medications.
- Be clear in your communication. Be honest and transparent with your doctor. Do not hold back any information. It is important that your doctor is aware of other treatment courses (other doctors, alternate medicines, stopping medications) that you may have been taking.
- Be on time for your appointments. At the same time, appreciate that the doctor is likely to be called away on emergencies or take longer time with patients who may have serious problems.

> - Do not crowd the clinic or hospital. Take only one attendant or family member with you, unless more are absolutely needed.
> - Be clear about financial issues with the hospital. Let the doctor know if there are constraints. This will help avoid hassles later.
> - If you have received good care, be lavish in your praise. Let the hospital and doctor know that you appreciate the work they have done for you.

I hope that these points will help you in getting the best care possible. I wish you and your loved ones a long and healthy life.

Acknowledgements

I owe a huge debt of gratitude to my dear friend and motivator-in-chief for this book, Dr Humeira Badsha. From the time I discussed the idea of writing this book, she has been my chief prodder, urging me to take it one chapter at a time, pushing me to focus on completing the book and chiding me when I dropped the ball, sometimes for weeks together. Suffice to say, without her, this book would possibly never have been completed.

My sincere thanks go to Rashmi T.K., who did most of the research for the book and who greatly helped me in putting the book together. She has been extremely patient and has persevered over all the time it took us to complete the book. Thanks also to Rohan Krishnan Alexander and Harikrishnan Warrier, who worked closely with Rashmi on the research for the book.

My thanks go to my family, especially my parents and two sons, who have always been my pillars of support.

My gratitude to all those who over the years have shared their experiences with the Indian healthcare system, the various experts who agreed to be interviewed for this book, my many colleagues who spoke to me in confidence, and to the innumerable patients whose experiences have helped shape this book. I also thank the beta readers who gave their feedback and helped make this book more reader-friendly.

To my publisher HarperCollins, Senior Commissioning Editor Bushra Ahmed, and my literary agent Anish Chandy of Labyrinth—a big thank you for all your support.

I hope this book will be the wake-up call that the Indian healthcare system needs and that policymakers and the healthcare industry will take concrete steps to correct the situation. Every Indian will certainly hope so once they read this book.

References and Notes

The detailed references and notes pertaining to this book are available on the HarperCollins *Publishers* India website. Scan this QR code to access the same.

About the Author

Dr Sumanth C. Raman, after graduating with an MBBS from Madras Medical College, worked as a consultant physician in Chennai, obtaining his M.D. in Internal Medicine along the way. His interests in the broader aspects of healthcare led him to work with Tata Consultancy Services as a key member of their Healthcare Innovation team.

A recognized thought-leader, Dr Raman regularly speaks on healthcare at national and international conferences. He is a well-known television personality and has over twenty-five years of medical experience; he has anchored over 3,000 programmes across various international, national and regional channels and is a regular part of television media debates. He writes articles on health, politics and social issues in several national newspapers and various national and international journals.

Dr Sumanth has previously authored the GK Smart Series of Books.

For more information, visit www.sumanthraman.com.